Psychiatry Interrogated

Bonnie Burstow
Editor

Psychiatry Interrogated

An Institutional Ethnography Anthology

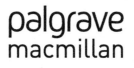

Editor
Bonnie Burstow
Ontario Institute for Studies in Education
University of Toronto
Toronto, Ontario, Canada

ISBN 978-3-319-41173-6   ISBN 978-3-319-41174-3   (eBook)
ISBN 978-3-319-42473-6 (softcover)
DOI 10.1007/978-3-319-41174-3

Library of Congress Control Number: 2016956475

Printed on acid-free paper

Cover design by Samantha Johnson

This Palgrave Macmillan imprint is published by Springer Nature
The registered company is Springer International Publishing AG
The registered company is Gewerbestrasse 11, 6330 Cham, Switzerland

This book is dedicated to everyone everywhere who has ever fallen prey to institutional psychiatry.

ACKNOWLEDGMENTS

I would like to acknowledge the hard work, the kindness, and the dedication of the various people who made this book possible—first and foremost my fellow authors Simon Adam, Joanne Azevedo, Rebecca Ballen, Chris Chapman, Agnieszka Doll, Mary Jean Hande, Efrat Gold, Sarah Golightley, Sonya Jakubec, Jennifer Poole, Janet Rankin, Lauren Spring, Sharry Taylor, Lauren Tenny, Jemma Tosh, Rob Wipond, and Eric Zorn. From the moment those heady workshops began in the summer of 2014, what a glorious adventure we have been on together! Thanks, Simon Adam and Brenda LeFrançois, for your initial recruitment work. I would likewise like to acknowledge the help of my tireless Palgrave editors, Rachel Krause and Elaine Fan, and my ever-vigilant graduate assistants—Sona Kazemi, Griffin Epstein, Lauren Spring, and Jan Vandertempel.

CONTENTS

Contributors

Simon Adam is a PhD candidate at the Ontario Institute for Studies in Education at the University of Toronto and teaches undergraduate nursing in Toronto. His academic and activist work center around the area of critiques of mental health and institutional analysis.

Joanne Azevedo is a PhD student at York University's School of Social Work. With more than two decades of frontline practice experience in child welfare, Joanne has a particular interest in critical race studies, feminist political economy, and discourse analysis.

Rebecca Ballen is a long-time antipsychiatry activist and an MSW student at York University.

Bonnie Burstow is a philosopher, an Associate Professor at the Ontario Institute for Studies in Education at the University of Toronto, and an antipsychiatry theorist. Her works include: *Psychiatry and the Business of Madness, The Other Mrs. Smith, Psychiatry Disrupted, The House on Lippincott, Radical Feminist Therapy,* and *Shrink-Resistant.*

Chris Chapman is an Assistant Professor, School of Social Work, York University, and is coeditor of *Disability Incarcerated: Imprisonment and Disability in the United States and Canada* (Palgrave Macmillan, 2015). He is coauthor of the forthcoming *Interlocking Oppression and the Birth of Social Work.*

Agnieszka Doll is a socio-legal researcher and lawyer. She is currently completing her PhD at the Law and Society Program, Faculty of Law, University of Victoria in Canada. She was called to the bar in Poland in 2005.

Efrat Gold is an independent researcher who holds an MA from the University of Toronto. Her interests include antipsychiatry/psychiatric survivors, feminist theory and practice, and creative resistance.

Sarah Golightley works for the Population Health Research Institute, University of London, where she researches mental health peer support. Her background is as a social worker and activist who has focused on antioppressive practice and LGBTQ+ support.

Mary Jean Hande is a doctoral candidate in Adult Education and Community Development at University of Toronto. She is committed to antipoverty and disability organizing.

Sonya L. Jakubec, RN, PhD is a community mental health nurse and researcher who employs critical, qualitative, and participatory research approaches. She is an Associate Professor with the School of Nursing and Midwifery in the Faculty of Health, Community and Education at Mount Royal University, Canada.

Jennifer Poole is an Associate Professor in the School of Social Work at Ryerson University. She brings all things "mad" and intersectional to her pedagogy, practice, research, and service both in and out of the academy.

Janet Rankin, PhD RN is a member of the Faculty of Nursing at the University of Calgary. Her research, using institutional ethnography, focuses on the impacts of hospital restructuring and health care reforms on nurses and patients.

Lauren Spring is a PhD candidate at the University of Toronto. Her research is focused primarily on arts-based approaches to consciousness-raising and working with survivors of trauma. Lauren is also the Creative Director of Extant Jesters (www.extantjesters.com).

Sharry Taylor is a high school teacher in Toronto, Ontario. She has an MEd from the Department of Leadership, Higher and Adult Education at the Ontario Institute for Studies in Education, University of Toronto.

Lauren Tenney, PhD, MPhil, MPA is a psychiatric survivor and activist, first involuntarily committed to a psychiatric institution at age 15. Her academic and media work aims to expose the institutional corruption, which is a source of profit for organized psychiatry, and to abolish state=sponsored human rights violations (www.laurentenney.us).

Jemma Tosh is a Research Manager in the Faculty of Health Sciences at Simon Fraser University and a Postdoctoral Research Fellow at the Institute for Gender, Race, Sexuality and Social Justice at the University of British Columbia. She is the author of *Perverse Psychology* and *Psychology and Gender Dysphoria*.

Rob Wipond has been a freelance magazine journalist and social commentator for two decades. He has received a number of journalism and magazine awards for his writings related to the social politics of psychiatry.

Eric Zorn holds a master's degree in Adult Education and Community Education at the University of Toronto, Ontario Institute for Studies in Education. His research is focused on how adult literacy programs meet the needs of learners who have experienced trauma and violence.

LIST OF FIGURES

CHAPTER 1

Introduction to the Project: IE Researchers Take on Psychiatry

Bonnie Burstow

What you have in your hands is a relatively static object—a book. You picked it up, perhaps, because something in the title piqued your interest. Even though you can, metaphorically speaking, engage in conversations with it, nonetheless it belongs on some level to the category of "things." That said, no book is "just a thing." Every book was once upon a time a book project. Every book required people to perform certain tasks to bring it into existence. Moreover, there was a reason for writing it; there was "knowledge" that one hoped to disseminate, create, validate, or even, in some instances, to mandate. Such is the nature of all book projects. At the same time, what underlays this specific one is a particularly multifaceted project that goes beyond the book, yet that is critical to understanding it.

As an entry point into this larger project, at this juncture I introduce you to a section of the very first document produced in relation to it. In the opening months of 2014, hundreds of people from various walks of life received a letter that read in part:

> Dr. Bonnie Burstow, Simon Adam, and Dr. Brenda LeFrançois invite you to become involved as a potential contributor in an exciting and original project. … Combining capacity-building and knowledge production, the project will culminate in an anthology of institutional ethnography (IE) pieces on psychiatry. Each contributor will be writing about a different aspect of the regime of ruling, perhaps also out of a specific disjuncture or problem that occurs to a specific population (e.g., trans, gay, "intellectually disabled," Aboriginal, women, children "in care"), and inevitably with respect to texts that are activated in a very

B. Burstow (✉)
Adult Education, Ontario Institute for Studies in Education, University of Toronto, Toronto, ON, Canada
e-mail: bonnie.burstow@utoronto.ca

© The Editor(s) (if applicable) and The Author(s) 2016
B. Burstow (ed.), *Psychiatry Interrogated*,
DOI 10.1007/978-3-319-41174-3_1

1

specific location (e.g., Quebec, British Columbia, New York, Poland, in the cells at Penetanguishene, in a nursing home in Bolivia). ... You have been contacted because we feel that you could contribute something unique and important. This may be on the basis of past IE work. Alternatively, it may be on the basis of your expert critical knowledge of psychiatry. In this regard, this is a two-pronged project: a) providing IE training to people who are interested but lack the necessary IE knowledge, and b) producing an anthology. As such, it is an opportunity for old hands at IE to apply their well-honed skills to critiquing psychiatry, and for old hands at critiquing psychiatry to at once produce a stunning piece of work and acquire a handy new skill. (Burstow, Adam, and LeFrançois, personal correspondence with prospective contributors)

The document went on to invite those interested to a series of four free workshops (five-and-a-half days in total), three of which were to help people acquire or hone "institutional ethnography" skills (as well as to help them get started on their own particular research project), and one explicitly devoted to helping participants "unhook from psychiatry." With this, possible contributors found their entry point into the project. And with this, we have our entry point into this book.

This book contains a series of institutional ethnography inquiries into psychiatry. This being the introduction, by the time this chapter ends, you will have a good idea about what you will find in this book—that is, what themes run through it, what each chapter covers or attempts to make visible, what institutional ethnography (IE) itself is, why IE is being applied to psychiatry, and what the purpose of the book and the project are. Systematically, making all this visible and intelligible,[1] such is the work of this chapter.

To begin with the last of these, for we have already dipped into these waters, as suggested in the foregoing, the purpose of this book and the project underlying it is: (1) to shed a critical light on psychiatry and (2) to bring the power of institutional ethnography to bear in the process. In addition, the purpose of the project per se is to help those critically aware, especially those already involved in antipsychiatry or "mad" activism, to acquire a highly serviceable new tool with which to expose psychiatry; and also to swell the ranks of psychiatry's able critics by attracting old hands at IE into the area. The book, in this regard, is both an educational product and a way of injecting new life into a liberatory movement.

WHY "TAKE ON" PSYCHIATRY?

Those of us who have been studying, combatting, and writing about psychiatry for years have little trouble answering the question posed in the heading, why "take on" psychiatry? Although psychiatry may seem like a lifeline to some and though its tenets and approaches have become so hegemonic—so like the air we breathe—that it may even seem counterintuitive to question them, as a critical mass of survivors have testified for decades now (e.g., see Fabris 2011) and as able critics have repeatedly demonstrated, psychiatry is a fundamentally problematic institution. For one thing, it rips people out of their lives and whatever may or may not have been bothering them earlier; suddenly, they find themselves with a serious new problem—they have little or no control over their daily existence. A statement made by an interviewee during one of my research projects fully exemplifies this dimension:

> So I'd mouthed off! Not ideal, I agree, but it was nothing. It's not as if other guys haven't done something similar from time to time, and it's not as if there was no provocation. My co-worker, he had just made fun of my work, and like, I'm sensitive about stuff like that. Anyway, I go back to my desk. Then I start getting ready to take off for lunch when this ambulance pulls up. Seriously! And before I know it, these two men, they have me in restraints and are taking me to hospital. Anyway, we arrive at the hospital and I try to explain that some sort of mistake has been made, but this nurse is asking me these questions that make no sense to me. Then they are pumping these drugs into me—and I have no say whatever— drugs which are making it impossible for me to think straight, even to stand. And a couple of days later, maybe a week, they are telling me that my regular ways of handling conflict are but a few of the many symptoms of this disease that I have, also that I probably have to stay on these medications for life. Anyway, for two long months, I am forced to stay in this place, all the while staff insisting I take these meds, watching my every move, telling me where to go, what to do, and, like, calling almost all of my actions symptoms. Now finally, they release me. But the thing is, I am still on these meds—and these workers, they keep turning up at my home to ensure that I am continuing to be what they call "treatment compliant." So I have to ask, just what has happened to my independence? What has happened to my life? (interview with Lucas—pseudonym used)

What we see here, at the very least in part, is control being presented as "treatment." This story, I would add, is hardly unique. Nor is what has surfaced here the totality of what is wrong with this institution.

Difficult though it may be to wrap one's head around this, there is additionally something profoundly wrong with psychiatry "medically," also on what might be called the hermeneutic level. As shown by Breggin (1991), Whitaker (2010), Woolfolk (2001), and Szasz (1987), there is no valid science underlying psychiatry, no proof that a single one of these putative diseases arise from a chemical imbalance—this despite years of insisting that they do—nor indeed proof that *any physical correlate of any sort* exists. Nor do their categorization schema (e.g., diagnoses) hold any explanatory value—for they are intrinsically circular (in this last regard, see Burstow 2015, Chapters 4 and 5). To quote from an interview with me in this regard:

> **LS:** You refer in your book to the DSM [*Diagnostic and Statistical Manual of Mental Disorders*] as a "boss text." Could you elaborate?
> **BB:** As a central text, it sets practitioners up to look at distressed and/or distressing people in certain ways. So, if they go into a psychiatric interview, they're going to be honing in on questions that follow the logic of the DSM, or to use their vocabulary, the "symptoms" for any given "disease" they're considering. In

the process it rips people out of their lives. And so now there's no explanation for the things people do, no way to see their words or actions as meaningful because the context has been removed. In essence, the DSM decontextualizes people's problems, then re-contextualizes them in terms of an invented concept called a "disorder."

I proceed by offering the following example. "Selective mutism," I begin:

…is a diagnosis given to people who elect [to] not speak in certain situations. So, if I were a non-psychiatrist—that is, your average thinking person who is trying to get a handle on what's going on with somebody—I would try to figure out what situations they aren't speaking in, try to find out if there's some kind of common denominator, to ascertain whether there's something in their background or their current context that would help explain what they are doing. You know, as in: Is it safe to speak? Is this, for example, a person of color going silent at times when racists might be present? Alternatively, is this a childhood sexual abuse survivor who is being triggered? Whatever it is, I would need to do that. But this is not what the DSM, as it were, prompts. In the DSM, "Selective Mutism" is a discrete disease. So, *according to psychiatry,* what causes these "symptoms" of not speaking? Well, "Selective Mutism" does. Note the circularity. That's what all the "mental disorders" are like: No explanatory value whatever. (Burstow and Spring 2015, p. XX)

Now for some—not me—even the circularity evident here might be acceptable if the "treatments" actually helped people. However, far from *correcting* imbalances—the "treatments" have been shown conclusively to *cause* imbalances (see Breggin 2008; Whitaker 2010). They also give rise to highly uncomfortable neurological diseases (see Breggin 2008). Moreover, evidence suggests that in the long run, irrespective of "diagnosis," people who were never once on these substances fare better than people who either stay on them or use them for a short time (see Whitaker 2010; Burstow 2015). Put all this together, and what starts to become clear is that framing what is happening as "help" is at the bare minimum suspect.

By everyday standards, this is harm. Which is not to say that individual psychiatrists are never helpful to people—only that the evidence suggests that psychiatry overall does far more harm than good. People end up hooked on brain-damaging drugs for life. People end up losing the multifaceted life that they once knew. Indeed, as Foucault (1980) and Burstow (2015) suggest and, as Lucas's words exemplify, what is being called help would appear to be little more than control. Nor is that the whole of the story.

Probe further and what you find, as demonstrated by Whitaker (2010), Burstow (2015), and Whitaker and Cosgrove (2015), whatever else may be involved, vested interests underlying and associated with psychiatry are blatantly driving this pathologization agenda—whether it be those of the multinational pharmaceutical enterprises or those of the American Psychiatric Association (which alas, at this point are close to identical). That is, interests are being served that are far from those of the people hypothetically being helped—all the while with the aid of claims that do not stand up to scrutiny and explanations that are circular. Still, psychiatry as an institution continues to wield incredible power—including the power to invalidate people's words, to drum people out of their professions (see Chapter 3), and to incarcerate people who have committed no crime. Moreover, firmly ensconced as an agent of the state, it continues to grow by leaps and bounds; and it continues to enjoy widespread credibility. The average person, that is, accepts the "knowledge" that it "mandates," the terms that it employs, the power that it wields. As such, anything that can help the average person step back and acquire a different view of psychiatry is a task worth doing.

WHY INSTITUTIONAL ETHNOGRAPHY?

Which brings us to the pivotal question: Yes, whether we view psychiatry as something to be discarded or something to be reformed—and to be clear, the various contributors to this book have different positions on this question—psychiatry needs to be "interrogated." That in itself, however, does not explain why the initial instigators of this project, and why the many more who flocked to it, were so keen to bring an IE perspective to bear—for clearly it is the institutional ethnography focus that most distinguishes this book and this project. What has IE to offer? What have IE researchers to contribute that is not found, say, in the brilliant works by Foucault (1980), Szasz (1961, 1970, 1987), or Breggin (2008)?

The answer to these questions lies in what institutional ethnography as an approach is all about—how it is conceived, what is involved, what it is uniquely positioned to bring to light.

INTRODUCING INSTITUTIONAL ETHNOGRAPHY

Significantly, no one versed in IE could have read the discussion of problems posed by psychiatry, as elucidated in the last few paragraphs, without "recognizing" that they were in quintessential IE territory—for the entire description has, as it were, "institutional ethnography" written all over it. So what exactly is institutional ethnography? The brain-child of Dorothy Smith, IE is an alternate way to "do sociology" (see Smith 1987), or to put this another way, a unique approach to conducting research. To elucidate a few distinctions between mainstream sociology and IE, while mainstream sociology is inhabited with abstractions, such as "society" or "roles," IE investigators rigorously avoid abstractions, sticking instead with the concrete "doings" of people. And while most sociologists operate in terms of the sociological literature (i.e., finding the research questions from them and understanding what they come across through that lens), IE investigators' reference point is the everyday world.

Institutional ethnography is a type of ethnography, but as the name suggests, it is particularly aimed at ferreting out and making visible how institutions work. Unlike with traditional ethnographies, correspondingly, which stay within the local to explain local phenomena (for a traditional ethnography, see Spradley 1979), a guiding principle of IE is that critical though the local is, local problems cannot be understood by investigating the local only for regimes "rule" centrally, from what Smith calls "elsewhere and elsewhen" (see Smith 1987, 2005, 2006; Smith and Turner 2014).

To use the example of Lucas, if we restricted ourselves to the local, we would know, in general, that he was wrested from his life. We would know who picked him up, where he was taken, and what was done to him. We would not know, however, on what authority, how it is that something called "an ambulance" comes to pick someone up on the basis of what would appear to be fairly innocuous actions. Nor why one drug and not another. Nor from whence came either the pathologizing or the drug imperative.

If some of the concepts touched on to date sound familiar, it should be noted that IE has been profoundly influenced by specific movements and specific schools of thought of which you may be knowledgeable (e.g., the women's movement(s), standpoint theory, Marxism, ethnomethodology). To go through a number of these, beginning with the women's movement, from her experiences in that movement, Smith concluded that despite claims to universality, sociology, and indeed, all disciplines reflect the standpoint of men and systematically leave out and/or distort the reality of women. She generalized to other oppressed groups—thus the centrality of standpoint theory (to be discussed shortly). She incorporated from Marxism the commitment to tying everything to the materiality of our existence—additionally the kind of direction that comes from taking seriously such queries by Marx and Engels (1973, p. 30) as: "Individuals always started, and always start, from themselves. Their relations are the relations of their real life. How does it happen that their relations assume an independent existence over [or] against them. And that the forces of their li[ves] overpower them?" Think back to Lucas's question, "What has happened to my life?" and you begin to get the relevance.

Correspondingly, drawing on ethnomethodology (see Garfinkel 1967), Smith asserts that society is not a phenomenon with an independent existence, not an agent capable of action, but something in motion, something continually created and recreated through the concrete "work" of people as they go about their everyday lives. By way of example, should you and I enter a conversation, then stop because someone has just approached, saying, "Excuse me," all three of us are together bringing into being the social. Some concrete IE terms that I would introduce at this juncture are: "disjuncture," "standpoint," "entry point," "problematic," "regime of ruling," "ruling," "regulatory frame," "textual mediation," "boss texts," "mapping," and "institutional capture."

Institutional ethnography research is intrinsically concerned with what IE researchers call "regimes of ruling" (Smith 1987, 2006). Pragmatically speaking, how can you identify a specific complex as a ruling regime (also sometimes referred to as a "knowledge regime")? One way is by the power that it wields, together with the privileged discourse that it employs—discourse that presents itself as "knowledge" and that determines how people and actions are viewed. An example is the criminal justice system, together with words such as "crime," "infraction," "disturbance of the peace," and "officer of the law." Other examples are every single academic "discipline." Additionally, you can hypothesize a "ruling regime" when things are happening at the local level that overwhelmingly serve the interests of extra-local conglomerates. An example of obvious relevance to this project is people staggering around from mandated drugs, with the benefit accruing to the multinational pharmaceutical companies.

All institutional ethnographies eventually come to focus on a regime of ruling. This, however, is not where inquiry begins. All begin locally in the everyday lives of people. More specifically, IE inquiries begin with a disjuncture—a break or fissure in the person's life or people's lives. It is present corporeally, engages her or his bodily existence. On a simple level, maybe a mother has taken her children to their local park to play, to her astonishment, only to find a bulldozed area where the park used to be (for an investigation that began with this very disjuncture see Turner 2014). Herein lies an "entry point."

Just as IE inquiries begin with a disjuncture, they begin with the adoption of a standpoint, almost invariably that of the person(s) experiencing said disjuncture. Here is where feminist standpoint theory enters in. Feminist standpoint theorists privilege women's standpoint over men's, and more generally, the standpoint of the oppressed over that of the oppressor, the claim being that the former allows people to see farther. It is not that theorists are maintaining that the standpoint of the oppressed yields "objective truth," for standpoint theorists to a person are clear that all knowledge is situated and partial (e.g., Harding 2004; Smith 2004). Only, in the words of standpoint theorist Nancy Hartsock (2004, p. 37), that it yields a vision "less partial" and "less perverse" (e.g., less harmful).

A clarification: "a standpoint" is not the same as a "perspective," and it is standpoint that is crucial to IE. It is not, that is, what the person experiencing the disjuncture believes, but what can be seen by standing in their position while on the alert for traces of institutional rule. If I might use a term put forward by standpoint theorist Nancy Hartsock (and to be clear, Hartsock means something much more extensive and communal in nature than what Smith has theorized), it is an "achieved standpoint." To understand this from within Smith's frame, it is the vision, that is, which the person would be capable of "achieving" if he or she theorized carefully from his or her own positionality and proceeded to investigate—a task that IE researchers take upon themselves.

Starting from the disjuncture and the related standpoint, the IE researcher proceeds to search for what is known in IE as a "problematic" (see Smith 2005, p. 38 ff.; Campbell 2002, p. 46 ff.). What is meant by the term "problematic"? Because this is one of those terms that befuddles most people, I would stick with a fairly instrumental answer. It is a particular kind of puzzle that presents itself. Problematics are a line of inquiry that holds the promise of opening up the ruling regime; in essence, rendering the disjuncture and what surrounds it "researchable." By way of example, in Chapter 2, you will be introduced to a research project in which the researchers start with the disjuncture of people being horrified by the sudden appearance of an advertisement recruiting individuals for an electroconvulsive therapy (ECT) experiment. How could this have happened? shock survivors asked. Pondering this enigma and wanting a line of inquiry that does not get stuck in individual psychology but is institutional in nature, the researchers proceeded to think of the "ethical review processes" that all proposed research must pass. They subsequently chose as the "problematic" how it is that the local Research Ethics Board authorized such a study and no higher authority in the ethical review hierarchy stopped it.

Armed with the disjuncture and a sense of the problematic, the IE researcher now "researches up"—that is, starts penetrating the various levels of the institution. With the understanding that in the modern era, ruling characteristically proceeds through centrally created texts, or, as IE puts it, is "textually mediated," the researcher is on the lookout for key texts. The focus, however, is not on texts in isolation but rather on relevant text–act sequences. How, for example, texts inform people's actions, which in turn are validated by those very texts. Questions explored include: Which institutional agent picks up which text? What do they do with it? Who do they pass it on to next? And, which other texts does it link up with? While all relevant levels of "textual mediation" are explored, of special significance are "boss texts"—texts high in the hierarchy on which lower subsidiary texts are modeled and/or in terms of which they function—for there is inevitably a textual hierarchy at play.

We have already come upon the concept of boss text—in the passage from my interview with Lauren Spring (LS) quoted earlier. Lauren, you recall, asked me about the emphasis that I put on the boss text in the DSM. In answering her question, I looked at one example of a diagnosis historically contained therein—Selective Mutism. What we saw from the example is that the text functions as a "regulatory frame" prompting the diagnostician to look for and to be prepared to find things called "symptoms" and to ignore everything else. As such, it legitimates what other institutional players proceed to do.

We noted the circularity—and indeed, circularity invariably characterizes institutional rule. The texts at once prompt the institutional players to look for certain qualities; willy-nilly, to "find" those qualities; to abstract those qualities from everything else in the person's life; and finally, at least in this case, to attribute them with causality. What causes the symptoms of not speaking in certain instances? In the world of the DSM, you will recall, "selective mutism" does. Now, although I did not cover this dimension in the interview, what makes a text such as the DSM a "boss text" is not only that it is frequently activated but also that subsidiary texts are modeled on it, with those additionally bringing the boss text into play—all the texts together engendering circularity.

A piece of research that demonstrates the circularity particularly clearly is George Smith (2014). The disjuncture? Police raiding the gay bathhouses in Toronto. On the everyday level, all that was happening before the meaning of the men's activities was reconstructed by the police was gay men pleasuring themselves. In his careful tracing of the text–act sequences, Smith demonstrates how this innocuous activity was constructed as a breaking of a law for which people could be charged.

The boss text being used by the police was the Bawdy House Law. The police entered a gay bathhouse with the intent of activating this text. As one section of the act[2] stipulates that a *bawdy house* is a place where people either buy sex or are engaged in "the practice of acts of indecency," the police were pointedly on the lookout for men, for instance, engaged in sexual acts behind booths whose doors were open—something, that is, that could be slotted under the category "acts of indecency." As another section of the law stipulates that any-one is liable to imprisonment of up two years in duration who is an "inmate" of a common bawdy house or *someone in control who knowingly permits this use of it*, they likewise focused in on the one worker present, observed what he saw—what his conduct could be construed as "knowingly" permitting.

The officer in charge proceeded to write up his "report" stating: "When the officers first entered the premises, they walked around noting … any *indecent activity*" [my emphasis, quoted from Smith 2014, p. 25], thereby drawing on the boss text definition of common "bawdy house." The officer then pointedly stated that there were people engaging in sex with the doors to their booths open. About the worker, he went on to write: "[DOE] walked past a number of rooms that were occupied by men [who] were masturbating themselves while others just lay on the mattress watching. At no time did [DOE] make an effort to stop these men or even suggest that they close the door to their booths" (quoted from Smith, p. 25)—an observation that fits, among other things, with the boss text term "knowingly permits the use of it," which in turn made DOE's actions or lack thereof actionable.

The point here is that the report, like the observation, was generated using the boss text categories, in other words, was so conceived as to "satisfy" the boss text criteria—which itself made what was transpiring "actionable." As such, the report led to charges against everyone. When, once again, all that was happening in the everyday world was gay men pleasuring themselves.

Smith (2014) diagrams the process, showing how it is put together, show-ing how the criminal code guides the observation, and how in turn the report fits with the sections of the criminal code and legitimizes the charges—all of it part of an ideological circle. This is precisely the kind of work that institutional ethnographers do—that is, what institutional ethnographers are able to show.

Generally, with the aid of visual diagrams, the institutional ethnographer "maps" the text–action sequences that enter into the ruling, unveils the circu-larity. In the process, she or he takes extra care not to get caught up in what IE calls "institutional capture"—that is, not to use the institution's words, concepts, ideology—but to stick with the disjuncture and concreteness of the text–act sequences, continuing to reach further and further into the extra-local so that all relevant levels are covered. In the process the researcher concretely demonstrates how the institution is, as it were, put together.

All well done IE research produces such understanding—thus, its value when addressing such hegemonic institutions as psychiatry, or what Parker (2014, p. 52) calls the "psy complex" (i.e., psychiatry, psychology, psychotherapy, psychiatric social work). All expose and provide ammunition for challenging.

One particular type of IE additionally makes activism integral to the methodology. Enter institutional ethnography George Smith-style—political activist ethnography—and, with a quick overview of it, I will end this depiction of IE.

George Smith, whose study of the bathhouse raids we just discussed, was a student of Dorothy's (no relation despite the same last name) and in what turned out to be a groundbreaking article, he articulated and provided us with concrete examples of how "grassroots activist IE research" could proceed (Smith 1990). In the unique approach to IE which he pioneered, research was in the service of activism, with the activist agenda at once dictating the research focus and functioning as the driving force that generates data. By way of example, in two separate studies, one challenging the bureaucracy's handling of the AIDS crisis, and the other, challenging the policing of the male gay community, he used not formal interviews but demonstrations and political face-offs to generate the data. He likewise used the documents that materialized in the defense of the people from the community being charged.

And, here we shift from institutional ethnography for understanding—albeit this variety can generate IE understanding that is every bit as intricate as the first—to institutional ethnography for social change. Other ways in which IE can culminate in social change include strategically using its findings for challenges and combining IE with activist approaches like participatory research.

Psychiatry, Institutional Ethnography, and the Historical Moment

The suitability of IE as an approach for interrogating psychiatry is demonstrable for psychiatry routinely causes disjunctures—indeed, horrendous disjunctures in people's everyday lives; it has both hegemonic and direct dictatorial power. Behind what we might initially see—a doctor or a nurse—lies a vast army of functionaries, all of them activating texts that originate extra-locally. The fact that IE as a method feels ready-made to unlock institutional psychiatry—and that's what I am suggesting here—is not accidental. Significantly, from early on, psychiatry was one of the primary regimes which Dorothy was theorizing as she went about developing her method.

Early pivotal works in this regard include: "K Is Mentally Ill" (Smith 1978), in which she examines the processes by which a woman is constructed as "mentally ill"[3]; "No One Commits Suicide" (Smith 1983), which explores the textual construction of suicide; and "Women and Psychiatry" (Smith 1975), which theorizes the special ruling of women. Now psychiatry has continued to be a focus in IE circles. Over time, nonetheless, it has become less central. One of the objectives of my previous book, *Psychiatry and the Business of Madness*, was to alter that dynamic.

With *Psychiatry and the Business of Madness* (Burstow 2015), the intent first and foremost was to write a psychiatry abolitionist text that would materially alter the landscape. At the same time—and these goals interpenetrated each other—it intended to use IE to open up psychiatry in a way that had not been done previously. In this regard, I wrote:

The strategic use of institutional ethnography is critical. … Even where IE as a methodology does not appear to be involved, as, say, in the history chapters, it is there in the background now guiding, now deepening the inquiry. *As such, IE serves not only as a primary methodology but as the overriding epistemology of the book.* IE, that is, is the lens through which we view all aspects of the institution, whether it be the relationship with the government, hospital texts, the nature of "prescribing," the very act of "diagnosing" … and the point is, ultimately, it is only by holding all such aspects together that we arrive at a grounded and comprehensive evaluation. That IE grounding in itself, I would add, separates this book from all other works on psychiatry, while opening up whole new ways of knowing. (Burstow 2015, pp. 20–21)

The intention was to bring institutional ethnography to bear on psychiatry in a new and powerful way while at the same time reasserting the significance of this area of investigation to the IE community itself.

At the point when I originally started envisioning the current anthology project, my earlier book was still under consideration by Palgrave Macmillan (later to be accepted and published). My thought as I approached possible coeditors for this anthology was that the first book (*Psychiatry and the Business of Madness*) could pave the way for the second (*Psychiatry Interrogated*). I envisioned it, as it were, as a "one-two punch." Moreover, I sensed, rightly or wrongly, partially as a result of the work of some of us and every bit as substantially because of the current groundswell of opposition to psychiatry, that we had arrived at a historical moment when psychiatry could once again be central to the IE world, and more significantly still, where an IE revolution in psychiatric critique was possible.

It is in this context that people were invited to take part in this one-of-a-kind anthology project. And it is in this context that excitement started to build.

Psychiatry Interrogated: The Process

To pick up on the story of the project where I left off pages ago, in the opening months of 2014 the three editors sent out a very large number of invitations, and many people signed on to the project, some with the intention of simply taking the training, others hoping to be a contributor. That noted, shortly after the first round of invitations went out, the other two editors withdrew.[4] Feeling the loss but determined to "soldier on," as sole editor and educator, I proceeded to plan and deliver the four workshops. Now a dilemma presented itself early on— how single-handedly to handle the logistics of the workshops, especially given that many participants would be attending virtually. The problem was quickly resolved when, thankfully, three graduate students (Eric Zorn, Efrat Gold, and Kelly Kay) offered to assist in exchange for being allowed to take the free IE training—a clear and early indication that, indeed, excitement over IE was brewing. All but one student subsequently became contributors to this book.

The formal training began July 7, 2014, and ended September 13, 2014. It took place at the Ontario Institute for Studies in Education (OISE). About three-fifths of the people attended virtually, while the rest were physically present. Major ingredients included: introduction to key aspects of IE; clarification of the project; and substantial experiential components where learners became skilled at recognizing institutional terms, at designing IE projects, at wrestling with problematics, at conducting interviews IE-style, and at mapping text–act sequences. Three components of particular note were: forming teams, beginning to draft projects, and the special workshop devoted to "unhooking" from psychiatry.

Identifying possible projects and the forming of teams occurred at the very last workshop. One reason that I opted for forming teams was that, given the huge turnout, we were in danger of having more research projects than could be easily accommodated in a single anthology. Another was that a transformative dimension enters in when research transpires communally. Although everyone, of course, created teams based on a common interest or passion, a configuration that I hoped would emerge were teams composed of both psychiatric survivors with expert knowledge of the institution but no knowledge of IE, on one hand, and skilled IE researchers who lacked the expert knowledge of the survivor on the other. A few such teams did indeed coalesce, and in each case, it was low on problems and high on mutual respect and synergy. By the end of the workshops, most contributors were part of a team.[5]

During the Unhooking from Psychiatry Workshop (the second to last one), it was clarified that people, of course, were *in no way obliged* to adopt an antipsychiatry position but they *were obliged* not to fall down into institutional capture. An example of an exercise we did in this regard involved dividing into small groups, with each one working through a list of words that reflect institutional capture—everyday terms (e.g., "mental illness," "mental health," "psychiatric diagnoses," and "psychiatric medication")—then brainstorming what might be used in their stead. The small groups subsequently presented to the group as a whole. I likewise shared my own recommendations, which are shown in Figure 1.1.

Now, while the exercise proceeded relatively seamlessly, of course, as most of us were well aware, it was one thing to be able to avoid institutional capture when part of a large group of people with one and only one task at hand—keeping psychiatry at bay. It was quite another when relatively on one's own and in the grip of other agendas. The question still to be answered was: What would happen when the research and the writing were in "full swing"?

The workshops ended with us all reaching out for ways to support each other and beginning the nitty-gritty of the work. Support groups formed. People talked in the hall. People exchanged email addresses. People told each other about documents that might be of use. People stepped up onto the advisory team. People checked in with me, wanting to ensure that what they were calling a "disjuncture" genuinely was one. Excitement was high, as was determination.

What followed over the next year was a flurry of activity, with researchers working away at problematics, hunting for documents, picking up threads and following them, searching for new threads, restructuring, checking in, and/or

Institutional Lingo	Possible non-institutional Replacements
has ADHD	Has been labeled ADHD
is schizophrenic	Labeled schizophrenic
mentally ill	Has or seen as having emotional difficulties
mental illness	Emotionally distraught
has history of mental illness	Has a history of being labeled "mentally ill"
family history of mental illness	Whole family is attributed as suffering from a "mental illness:
ward	I'd leave as is, but never forget that it is an institutional term
meds	drugs
medicated	Put on drugs
nurses	(I'd tend to leave it as is also—just don't forget it's an institutional category)
symptoms	Ways of being that others find distressing
psychiatric treatment	Psychiatric "treatment"
incapable of deciding on treatment issues	Labeled "incapable"
effective treatment	"treatment" claimed to be helpful
psychosis	Ways of being, thinking, or acting that others not understand
acted out	Acted in ways that staff did not like
hallucinations	Seeing or hearing things others do not hear or see
diagnosis	label
dual diagnosis	Two labels
committed to an institution	Psychiatrically incarcerate
suffered a relapse	Return to way of acting or thinking that was defined as a problem
noncompliant	Actively rejects what the "mental health" professional asks of him/her

Figure 1.1   An example of material looked at during the September 12, 2014, workshop: Beginning to Think About How to Unhook From Psychiatric Discourse

altering the focus. Driven by a passion, generally related to the disjuncture that they so keenly felt, for several months various teams remained on the lookout for people external to the anthology project who were concerned about the same problem; the same disjuncture; and when it felt right, proceeded to blend them into the team, with some teams growing exponentially in the process. Even though some projects dropped out—and we all particularly regretted the disappearance of three projects in the Indigenous and Aboriginal areas—most teams continued, delighted by the knowledge that they were generating, and indeed, eager to share it. A development of special note in this regard is that long before this anthology was written or even under consideration by the publisher, already a large number of the contributors had presented findings of their research at academic conferences.

The stellar researchers and authors of Chapter 3 (Chris Chapman, Jennifer Poole, Rebecca Ballen, and Joanne Azevedo), for example, were investigating how the regulated professions psychiatrically monitor their own practitioners. At that time none of the team members had previous IE experience. Nonetheless, individually and collectively, within nine months, each and every member of the team had presented findings at multiple conferences, with all presentations/papers enthusiastically received.[6] The fact that this team was so early to bring its findings to the world, that the research was so well received, that the team intends to continue their work together long after this anthology is out—indeed, will be leveraging its ongoing findings to challenge the pathologizing/oppressive practices of the "regulated professions"—what more could one ask? That is precisely the kind of engagement that an editor dreams will materialize when initiating a project of this ilk.

While there have already been too many exciting developments to list, one that especially warms my heart, and that I cannot but reference in passing, is the work of a team of 15 American psychiatric survivors—all honing in on the pathologizing of spirituality (see Chapter 4). While Lauren Tenney is the sole author of the chapter and while at the time of penning this introduction, this team's research proposal remained in the drafting stage, significantly, its work is also continuing. Correspondingly, what is happening here realizes in a very tangible way one of the primary objectives of the project: making IE skills available to psychiatric survivors.

Note too, in this regard, that only one "member" "officially" joined the book project and attended the workshops—Lauren. Nonetheless, drawing on work that they had done together earlier, she proceeded to gather around her a very large team of fellow psychiatric survivors (some use other descriptors), all of whom she helped acquire IE skills. Many are continuing the project with her, and several provided major input for Chapter 4—something that in my culture we call a "mitzvah." I would add here that the vast majority of those who joined teams in the period *between the end of the workshops and the submission of the chapters* were psychiatric survivors—again, a gratifying development.

That noted, to give you a sense of the general process from the perspective of a member of one of the teams, scholar Jennifer Poole (personal correspondence) writes:

> It was Bonnie who brought us together first, inviting me (Jennifer), Chris and Rebecca to participate in this IE book project. We met at OISE last summer with folks from near and far, and began to share our ideas for possible chapters. I had been long concerned with the "reporting" of friends and colleagues in social work for reasons related to their "mental health." I feared the "discipline" and "distress" subsequently visited on those friends and how soon it would be visited on me. Speaking [of] this fear in the group, Chris nodded, so did Rebecca and we started to discuss being a "team." At a hearing for one of those friends months later, I shared our work to date with Joanne, also sitting in support. She was interested too, and after a nod from Chris and Rebecca, our team was born and the planning began. Six months later, we have conducted a REB-approved research

pilot, presented five papers at two conferences and are working towards project specific funding and hopefully, policy change. This chapter is just the beginning.

Did any of the teams fall into institutional capture as feared? Indeed, at various points and to varying degrees, the majority did. In some cases, this was because the researchers' own location as members of the ruling regime made navigating the terrain especially tricky—a kind of double bind that it might have been helpful to have given more thought to when constructing the "Unhooking from Psychiatry" workshop. In most, it was simply because of the pervasive hegemony of the institution—a lesson in itself on how very difficult it is for people to "unhook" from psychiatry even under optimal conditions. That said, people plowed on. People rethought and rewrote.

And, in the fullness of time, a truly exceptional anthology materialized.

Psychiatry Interrogated: The Journeys, the Chapters

Penetrating, eye-opening, the book, the various journeys, the chapters that lay ahead of you are each and every one the product of extensive research—all of it compelling, all of it breaking new ground, all of it drawing on IE to varying degrees. In some cases, the inquiry is almost exclusively IE in nature (e.g., Doll, Chapter 10). In others, it is combined with additional types of inquiry, whether it be traditional historical research (Gold, Chapter 11) or some combination of critical discourse analysis and participatory research (Tenney, Chapter 4). In some, IE is used methodologically (e.g., Burstow and Adam, Chapter 2), while in others it serves more as an epistemology (Spring, Chapter 7). Some chapters focus more directly on psychiatry (Burstow and Adam, Chapter 2; Spring, Chapter 7), while others zero in on other parts of the psy complex, or one of the cognate disciplines,[7] or an intersecting discipline, whether it be nursing (Chapters 3 and 6), "mental health" lawyering (Chapter 10), social work (Chapter 8), psychology (Chapters 8 and 11), or the psychiatric ruling that occurs from within another major institution (e.g., the military—see Spring, Chapter 7).

Whereas some are more global in focus (Jakubec and Rankin, Chapter 6), most focus in on some country, some province or state, in one case, initially, on a single psychiatric institution (Burstow and Adam, Chapter 2). The specific geographical jurisdictions featured include: British Columbia (Wipond and Jakubec, Chapter 9), Manitoba (Gold, Chapter 11), the United States (Tenney, Chapter 4), Canada (Burstow and Adam, Chapter 2), Poland (Doll, Chapter 10), the United Kingdom (Tosh and Golightley, Chapter 8), and Ontario (Chapman, Poole, Ballen, and Azevedo, Chapter 3).

Each of the pieces of research carves out its own unique territory, allows us entry into a hitherto relatively unexplored corner of psychiatry. In addition, each maps out that corner in intricate detail (generally with the aid of highly revealing diagrams), and as such, each constitutes a formidable contribution to critical/antipsychiatry scholarship in its own right—also, as the case may be, to scholarship in such areas as military trauma, nursing, and social work. None of these chapters attempts to set forth the regime of ruling in its entirety, as, for example, happens in Burstow (2015). This notwithstanding, as you proceed from one chapter to the next, much like an infant fresh to the world, you begin to pick up a sense of the whole. This is largely because of the breadth, the diversity, the commonality of the approach, the reappearance of boss texts, the felt sense that travels from one chapter to another, and the overlapping themes.

In this last regard, various themes weave in and out of the chapters. Expectable themes that can be found in the majority of them include interference, trauma, violence, lives reduced to shambles. Other dominant themes, some that are expectable, some that may surprise you, include: the diagnostic folly of the DSM (Chapters 5 and 7), financialization (Chapters 5, 6, 9, and 11), the psy disciplines and the military (Chapters 7 and 11), the degradation of research (Chapters 2, 6, and 11), psychiatry and the workplace (Chapters 3, 8, 9, and 10), psychiatrization and poverty (Chapters 2, 5, and 6), globalization (Chapters 5 and 6), the psychiatric monitoring to which members of the regulated professions are subjected (Chapters 3 and 8), organized resistance (Chapters 2 and 4), and the treacherous relationship between doing the best possible for oneself or one's kin and falling into institutional capture (Chapters 5 and 7).

CHAPTER BY CHAPTER

At this juncture, you have more than a passing familiarity with this chapter. In ending, the following will give you a glimpse into each of the other chapters.

If ever you have placed faith in the integrity of the research done in academia or the processes that "monitor" it, Chapter 2 ("Stopping CAMH: An Activist IE Inquiry") will be an eye-opener. The one and only George Smith-style inquiry in this collection, authored by Burstow and Adam, this study involves an activist group, a formal complaint, and one of the largest psychiatric institutions in North America (Centre for Addictions and Mental Health or CAMH). The initial disjuncture was the sudden appearance of an alarming advertisement. Under the category "Jobs Etc." CAMH had placed an ad on Craigslist that in essence functioned so as to lure those down on their luck to be participants in an electroshock study—a study that involved them actually receiving ECT. In the battle and research that followed, hitherto hidden truths come to light not only about *psychiatric* research processes but, every bit as important, about research oversight in general.

Exquisitely written, Chapter 3 is called "A Kind of Collective Freezing-Out: How Helping Professionals' Regulatory Bodies Create Professional 'Incompetence' and Increase Pathologizable Distress." Herein Chapman, Poole, Ballen, and Azevedo use as an entry point into the institutional ruling the process by which two able nurses were declared "unfit to practice." The researchers trace the construction of these practitioners as "unfit," showing at the same time the conflation of "mental illness" with "incompetence." In one of the cases, they additionally suggest how anti-Black racist prejudices became deraced and reinscribed as incompetence as a result of "mental illness."

Chapter 4 ("Spirituality: A Participatory Planning Process") was penned by Tenney, with the backing of a large research team comprised of 14 other American psychiatric survivors. Each and every one was "psychiatrized" at least in part on the basis of what is, in essence, spiritual experiences. The very fact of this happening, the ripping of them out of their lives, the erasure of the spiritual—such is the disjuncture. How is it, asks Tenney, that nonhegemonic spiritual beliefs translate into a warrant for such profound interference?

Chapter 5 is the chapter that makes most visible the institutional capture fallen into by victims of the system. Called "Operation ASD: Philanthrocapitalism, Spectrumization, and the Role of the Parent" and authored by Hande, Taylor, and Zorn, it examines how parents of children diagnosed with autism become "captured" by the notion of the "Autism Spectrum Disorder." Correspondingly, the authors trace the social relations and text–action sequences that enter into the ASD diagnosis, beginning with the experiences of parents.

Chapter 6 is the sole chapter created exclusively by professionals who are themselves part of the regime of ruling. Authored by Jakubec and Rankin and titled "Interrogating the Rights Discourse and Knowledge Making Regimes of the 'Movement for Global Mental Heath'" (mGMH), it was written in the context of the "scaling up" of the "mGMH." Looking at a program that began benignly, the authors focus in particularly on what happens when a conflation occurs between people's rights being honored and their receiving of "psychiatric treatment."

Authored by Spring, Chapter 7 ("Pathologizing Military Trauma") begins with an enigma: Between 2004 and 2014, Canada lost more members of the Canadian Armed Forces to suicide than it did on the battlefield in Afghanistan. Now, the regime of ruling constructs these military suicides as a product of "mental illness" ("PTSD" especially). Correspondingly, public outcries for increased funding, "de-stigmatization" campaigns, and greater access to "professional treatment" abound. However, viewing and "treating" military trauma through the lens of psychiatry is profoundly damaging. Such is the disjuncture on which this chapter rests.

Written by Tosh and Golightley, Chapter 8, the one UK piece in this collection, is aptly named "The Caring Professions, Not So Caring?" It is made up of two case studies about bullying in UK universities, one involving a social work student, and the other, a faculty member in a psychology department; the initial disjuncture in one case occurring when a victim of bullying was labeled "mentally ill," and in the other, when someone was bullied because of a label of "mental illness." These two similar but opposing disjunctures offered an opportunity for comparative analysis, which the authors ably provide.

In Chapter 9 ("Creating a Better Workplace in Our Minds"), Wipond and Jakubec trace the construction of problems in the workplace as "mental health issues" and explore how legitimate grievances over workplace conditions are thereby neutralized. Singled out for special scrutiny is the "mental health continuum model."

In Chapter 10 ("Lawyering for the Mad"), Doll explores the double binds in which lawyers in Poland find themselves, demonstrating how the textual organization of legal aid appointments and the financing of legal aid representation relocates legal aid lawyering in commitment cases to the margins of lawyers' work. This, in turn, she shows, adversely affects the quality of legal representation received by those involuntarily institutionalized in psychiatric hospitals in Poland.

In the final chapter (Chapter 11), we return to the theme of the degradation of research. Many a reader will be familiar with the torturous experiments conducted by McGill psychiatrist Dr. Ewen Cameron. But did you know that torturous experiments were conducted as well by University of Manitoba psychologist John Zubek, also with links to the military? In "By Any Other Name," researcher Efrat Gold traces Zubek's immobilization research, its main funders, and their respective mandates—one of whom, curiously, was the enormously powerful US governmental body, the National Institute for Mental Health (NIMH). She additionally shows how the University of Manitoba structured these experiments as "ethical." Correspondingly, having drawn the parallel between the immobilization experiments and the current use of restraints in psychiatric institutions, she leaves us with the haunting question, "If not torture, what was NIMH's interest in Zubek's research?"

Following the final chapter is the "Afterword." It draws together where we have been. And it speculates on the implications for institutional ethnography itself. Urgent questions raised include: "What is lost—what sacrificed when we assume the standpoint of the frontline worker … somehow 'covers' … the standpoint of the 'patient'?"

Such then are the journeys that lay ahead.

NOTES

1. To be clear, I am in no way intending to equate the "visible" and the "intelligible." That said, visual representation is core to institutional ethnography—note, in this regard, the visual mapping.
2. For all referencing of the original documents, see Smith (1990, 2014).
3. For a more detailed discussion of this article, see Chapter 3.
4. One of the former coeditors, Brenda LeFrançois, went on to be an attendee at some of the workshops and for a while was part of a research team. Unfortunately, that team eventually dropped out because of life circumstances. The other former coeditor, Simon Adam, continued on in a contributor capacity and is coauthor, along with me, of Chapter 2. My thanks to both for the early work reaching out to potential contributors.
5. Four people opted to do solo projects. Of these, three indeed conducted the research and wrote up their chapters.
6. Papers presented include: "In Whose Interest? Un/fitness of Practice and the Ontario College of Social Workers and Social Service Workers" (presented by Azevdo, Ballen, Poole, and Chapman at a Canadian Disability Association conference, Ottawa, 2015); "Who Is Well Enough to Help Others? Interlocking

Oppressions, Compulsory Sound-Mindedness, and the Regulation of Helping Professionals" (presented by Chris Chapman at a Canadian Association of Social Work Educators conference, Ottawa, 2015); and "Duty to Report or Accommodate? Mental Health Disability, the AODA, and Social Work Now" (presented by Jennifer Poole, also at the conference of Canadian Association of Social Work Educators).

7. As in Burstow (2015), "cognate discipline" refers to nursing, psychology, and social work.

REFERENCES

Breggin, P. (1991). *Toxic psychiatry.* New York: St. Martins Press.

Breggin, P. (2008). *Brain-disabling treatments in psychiatry: Drugs, electroshock, and the psychopharmaceutical complex.* New York: Springer.

Burstow, B. (2015). *Psychiatry and the business of madness: An ethical and epistemological accounting.* New York: Palgrave.

Burstow, B., & Spring, L. (2015). Probing psychiatry and the business of madness. Retrieved on July 30, from http://rabble.ca/books/reviews/2015/07/probing-psychiatry-and-business-madness?utm_content=buffer0597f&utm_medium=social&utm_source=twitter.com&utm_campaign=buffer

Campbell, M. (2002). *Mapping social relations: A primer in doing institutional ethnography.* Aurora: Garamond Press.

Fabris, E. (2011). *Tranquil prisons.* Toronto: University of Toronto Press.

Foucault, M. (1980). *Power/knowledge* (C. Gordon, Trans.). New York: Pantheon.

Garfinkel, H. (1967). *Studies in ethnomethodology.* Englewood Cliffs: Prentice-Hall.

Harding, S. (Ed.) (2004). *The feminist standpoint reader* (pp. 35–53). New York: Routledge.

Hartsock, N. (2004). The feminist standpoint: Developing the grounds for a specifically feminist historical materialism. In S. Harding (Ed.), *The feminist standpoint theory reader* (pp. 35–53). New York: Routledge.

Marx, K., & Engels, F. (1973). *Feuerbach: Opposition of the materialist and the idealist outlooks.* London: Lawrence and Wishart.

Parker, I. (2014). Psychology politics resistance: Theoretic practice in Manchester. In B. Burstow, B. LeFrançois, & S. Diamond (Eds.), *Psychiatry disrupted* (pp. 52–64). Montreal: McGill-Queens University Press.

Smith, D. E. (1975). Women and psychiatry. In D. Smith & S. David (Eds.), *Women look at psychiatry* (pp. 1–19). Vancouver: Press Gang.

Smith, D. E. (1978). K is "mentally ill": The anatomy of a factual account. *Sociology, 12*(1), 23–53.

Smith, D. E. (1983). No one commits suicide: Textual analyses of ideological practices. *Human Studies, 6,* 309–359.

Smith, D. E. (1987). *The everyday world as problematic.* Toronto: University of Toronto Press.

Smith, D. E. (2004). Women's perspective as a radical critique of sociology. In S. Harding (Ed.), *The feminist standpoint reader* (pp. 21–33). New York: Routledge.

Smith, D. E. (2005). *Institutional ethnography: A sociology for people.* New York: AltaMira Press.

Smith, D. E. (Ed.) (2006). *Institutional ethnography as practice.* New York: Rowman and Littlefield.

Smith, D. E., & Turner, S. M. (Eds.) (2014). *Incorporating texts into institutional ethnographies*. Toronto: University of Toronto Press.

Smith, G. (1990). Political activist as ethnographer. *Social Problems, 37*(4), 629–648.

Smith, G. (2014). Policing the gay community: An inquiry into textually-medicated social relations. In D. E. Smith & S. Turner (Eds.), *Incorporating texts into institutional ethnographies* (pp. 17–40). Toronto: University of Toronto Press.

Spradley, J. (1979). *The ethnographic interview*. New York: Harcourt Brace Jovanovich College Publishers.

Szasz, T. (1961). *The myth of mental illness*. New York: Paul B. Hoeber.

Szasz, T. (1970). *The manufacture of madness*. New York: Harper and Row.

Szasz, T. (1987). *Insanity: The idea and its consequences*. New York: John Wiley and Sons.

Turner, S. (2014). Reading practices in decision processes. In D. E. Smith & S. M. Turner (Eds.), *Incorporating texts into institutional ethnographies* (pp. 197–224). Toronto: University of Toronto Press.

Whitaker, R. (2010). *Anatomy of an epidemic*. New York: Broadway Paperbacks.

Whitaker, R., & Cosgrove, L. (2015). *Psychiatry under the influence*. New York: Palgrave.

Woolfolk, R. (2001). The concept of mental of mental illness. *The Journal of Mind and Behavior, 22*, 151–187.

CHAPTER 2

Stopping CAMH: An Activist IE Inquiry

Bonnie Burstow and Simon Adam

A very curious institutional ethnography (IE) activist research project was kick-started in early August of 2012. The occasion? Surfing the net, psychiatric survivors and antipsychiatry activists and their allies found themselves faced with a profound disjuncture. An advertisement had appeared on Craigslist under the category "Jobs Etcetera" (entitled: Do You Suffer From Depression That Has Not Responded to Medication?—for the article in its entirety, see https:/drive.google.com/file/d/0B39eB1GoDYuQTjI0VG1GN2twX3M/edit?usp=sharing). An odd title for a job advertisement and a disjuncture in its own right.

The advertisement originated from researchers at the prestigious Centre for Addiction and Mental Health (CAMH) in Toronto. It was directed at long-term depressed people and given that it was placed in a category (Jobs Etcetera) that largely and predictably attracts two types of readers—those just wanting some extra money and those in dire need of it—and given the emphasis on what has been intractable depression, that it would be especially attractive to the latter was reasonably foreseeable, irrespective of whether the targeting of this group was actually intended. What was the "job"? Taking part in an allegedly comparatively safe research project that would involve undergoing a series of procedures—including (and such was the construction that this procedure looked minor) electroconvulsive therapy (ECT). The appearance of this advertisement constituted the research disjuncture.

B. Burstow (✉)
Adult Education, Ontario Institute for Studies in Education, University of Toronto, Toronto, ON, Canada
e-mail: bonnie.burstow@utoronto.ca

S. Adam
School of Nursing, Trent University, Peterborough, ON, Canada

B. Burstow (ed.), *Psychiatry Interrogated*,
DOI 10.1007/978-3-319-41174-3_2

21

How is it that a mental health center was reaching out into the general public for subjects for ECT experiments?—moreover, calling it "work" and portraying it as innocuous, people asked. How is it that recruitment of this nature could even be allowed? Duly alarmed, concerned individuals throughout North America sprang into action—and an engagement began that was to acquire a life of its own. It consisted of challenging the existence and the modus operandi of the study and in the process analyzing and exposing it. What was involved was at once engaged scholarship and more traditional activism. Activists and psychiatric survivors were at the forefront, especially members of Coalition Against Psychiatric Assault (CAPA). And as engaged or activist scholars, both of the authors of this chapter were centrally involved.

Emergent in its design, before long a full-scale activist-oriented IE research project coalesced, with Burstow (this chapter's first author) at the center of it, aimed at discovering how this could have happened and, more importantly insofar as possible, putting an end to it. What was identified in the process was a series of pivotal players, documents, and mechanisms, all of whose interactions and connections needed to be analyzed and understood—including the Centre for Addiction and Mental Health (CAMH), CAMH's Research Ethics Board (REB), the University of Toronto's (U. of T.) research ethics processes and oversight mechanisms, and the Secretariat on Responsible Conduct of Research. Correspondingly, one particular boss text quickly became focal—the Tri-Council Policy Statement (Canadian Institute of Health Research, Natural Sciences and Engineering Research Council of Canada, and Social Sciences and Humanities Research Council of Canada 2010).

The purpose of this chapter is to make sense of and to trace the activist research project in question and to elucidate the institutional processes surrounding the CAMH research as they came to light. As is standard in political activist ethnography (see Smith 1990)—and one of the major distinctions between this chapter and others in this anthology, the IE approach used was of the George Smith variety—activism informed the inquiry and the inquiry drove the activism. To put this in more familiar research language, data collection did not arise from conducting interviews and/or engaging in dedicated periods of observation but precisely in the activist attempt to effect change. In the process, mapping happened and discoveries were made.

What was discovered with respect to the operation of CAMH per se is a lack of transparency, both the use of boss texts and the circumvention of boss texts; moreover, circuits of accountability which, irrespective of intention, function overwhelmingly to mystify processes and prevent accountability. What was found with regard to federal research oversight in Canada, correspondingly, are accountability structures that, except in a very circumscribed area, are unable to protect; and, as such, constitute a disjuncture in their own right.

THE DISJUNCTURE AND THE INITIAL RESPONSE TO IT

The initial disjuncture was experienced by a number of the populations. These include researchers and scholars whose work demonstrates that ECT is damaging (e.g., Peter Breggin) and activists who had been organizing against ECT for decades. An even more pivotal population—and these groups greatly overlap—were psychiatric survivors, particularly ECT survivors, who were especially horrified. Here were people who had to take notes all day long because of the memory impairment caused by ECT. As such, their claim to know was grounded in the turbulence caused in their everyday lives. As they struggled from one day to the next to remember whom they talked to and what had been said, they found themselves staring in disbelief at an advertisement assuring people in need of money that receiving ECT was, in essence, a convenient way to make ends meet.

Survivors and activists were the first to act. Their work consisted in alerting everybody whom they thought might be able to address this situation. In this regard, survivors from across North America wrote directly to politically engaged and activist professionals, including Dr. Peter Breggin and Dr. Bonnie Burstow, and to activist groups. Before long, I (Burstow) personally and the one antipsychiatry group in the area—the Coalition Against Psychiatric Assault—had received numerous emails and telephone calls from people across the continent. "How can this be okay?" asked one stunned ECT survivor (L. Roberts [pseudonym], personal communication, August 10, 2012). "Can you or Don [fellow activist] do something about it?" asked another (Anonymous, personal correspondence, August 11, 2012). A few of us activists talked. What followed was a quick piece of cyber-activism. Individual activists and survivors urged the Craigslist site to remove the offensive advertisement. The action was successful. Of course, no one was under any illusion that removing the ad would stop either the problematic study or the problematic recruitment per se.

To understand the depth of the reaction one needs to take in that behind this disjuncture were decades of disjunctures—together with survivor testimony in response to it. Note, in this regard, as long as ECT has been in use, its survivors have experienced a profound disconnect between the official ECT line and their own experience—a reality that they were in no way prepared for when they either "consented" to electroshock or had it imposed on them. Although the official position is that it is safe and effective and that it involves only minor and transient memory loss (see Fink 1978, 1999, 2009), for example, what the lived experiences of a huge number tell us is that it creates extensive and permanent memory loss and that it in essence leaves one's life in shambles. Having experienced the profound disconnect firsthand, correspondingly, survivors repeatedly have drawn on their expert knowledge of ECT to publically challenge the official line. There are literally thousands of such pieces of testimony.

To get a flavor of what has been said, take a look at the testimony from the last Toronto hearing into ECT, the totality of which can be found at Inquiry into Psychiatry (2005). Similarly, witness this statement recently made by shock survivor Linda Andre:

> Imagine you wake up tomorrow with your past missing. ... You may not be able to recognize your home or know where your bank accounts are. ... You can't remember your wedding or your college education. Eventually you realize that years of your life have been erased, never to return. Worse, you find that your daily memory and mental abilities aren't what they were before. (Andre 2009)

Or witness this piece of public testimony delivered by ECT survivor Connie Neil decades earlier:

> I was ... studying playwriting. As anyone knows, the kind of creative writing that you do ... depends very strongly on what you are made up of, what your past memories are, your past relationships, how you deal with other people, how others deal with other people—all these things. I can't write any more. ... Since the shock treatment, I'm missing between eight and fifteen years of memory and skills; and this includes most of my education. I was a trained classical pianist. ... Well, the piano's in my house, but ... it just sits there. I don't have that kind of ability any longer. It's because when you learn a piece and you perform it, it's in your memory. But it doesn't stay in my memory. None of these things stay in my memory. People come up to me ... and they tell me about things we've done. I don't know who they are. I don't know what they're talking about, although obviously I have been friendly with them. Mostly what I had was ... modified shock, and it was seen as effective. By "effective," I know that it is meant that they diminish the person. They certainly diminished me. ... I work as a payroll clerk for the Public Works Department. I write little figures and that's about all. And it's a direct result of the treatment. (Phoenix Rising Collective 1984, 20A–21A)

To understand what the sudden appearance of the Craigslist advertisement meant to people on the ground, it is important to take into account the decades of suffering, the decades of "lived betrayal," and the clamoring for change, evidenced in the preceding. Correspondingly, it is vital to view the appearance of the advertisement through the eyes of survivors and those of us who have been keeping faith with survivors' experiences over the years. An inherently brain-damaging procedure (see Breggin 2007; Sackeim et al. 2007; Burstow 2015a) was being described as safe and effective. Psychiatric survivors who experienced their lives as having been stolen from them by this "treatment" were seeing ECT depicted as an utterly minor procedure and indeed a form of "work." Moreover, irrespective of intention, "vulnerable" (i.e., in ethical review terminology) people who may be in need of a few extra dollars were being "targeted"—people, significantly, who otherwise would have escaped this procedure, together with the damage that would inevitably ensue. The question then was not whether an objection was necessary. The question was *what* course of action to pursue.

We initially thought about demonstrating against CAMH. As those in the field were all well aware, however, demonstrations against psychiatric institutions almost never culminate in any kind of redress. Indeed, so common are they at this point that they do not even succeed in drawing attention to the issue.

THE STRUCTURE AND THE CHOICE OF DIRECTION

As we considered what to do, the boss text and the institutional research processes in which CAMH is embedded became focal. To introduce them at this juncture, CAMH is a huge and indeed prestigious psychiatric teaching hospital in the center of Toronto, affiliated with the University of Toronto. The significance of its being a teaching hospital is that it is subject to the institutional processes that govern all academic and hospital research in Canada. To get to the advertising stage—and at this juncture, clearly, it was well into that stage—the research in question was approved and necessarily had to have been approved by CAMH's Research Ethics Board. The power structures involved can be seen in Figure 2.1.

Witness the studies at the bottom of the figure and CAMH's REB right above it. Like all REBs in Canada, the CAMH one was set up in accordance with the direction of a specific boss text and in turn is regulated by that boss text—the Tri-Council Policy Statement (TCPS; also TPS). The TCPS itself is overseen by the Secretariat of Responsible Conduct of Research. Because all research conducted in Canada is accountable to this higher-up body, as all, moreover, are regulated by and are expected to adhere to the principles articulated in the Policy statement; ostensibly, there was an institutional way of challenging the CAMH research.

What was envisioned, accordingly, was placing a formal complaint with the Secretariat, articulating each misfit with the Policy Statement's principles. What was envisioned, in IE terms, was the use of a boss text precisely for *activist* purposes. This stands in sharp contrast with the typical activist route of a demonstration—the other option considered. We quickly chose the institutional option because of the failure of past demonstrations against CAMH to even garner press coverage.

The decision was initially made through an email exchange between CAPA activist Don Weitz and Bonnie Burstow. Having sat on a university REB and having had extensive experience with ethical review, Burstow was well positioned to lodge a complaint. She, accordingly, suggested that this route be prioritized. Don agreed. Others were asked, and within short order, all parties involved in the conversation had consented.

Examples of Relevant Sections from the TCPS

A number of the sections of the TCPS and a number of articulated values and principles therein are relevant to the complaint envisioned. The issue of harm is one of them. This is clearly articulated in TCPS 1, which states that

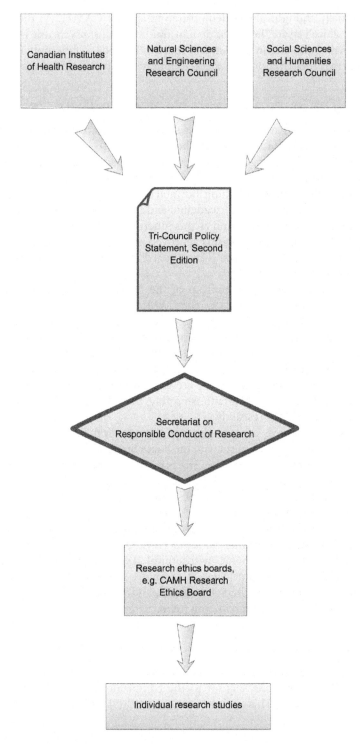

Figure 2.1   The Tri-Council hierarchy

there must be a favorable "harms–benefits balance" and further stipulates that "[r]esearch subjects must not be subjected to unnecessary risks or harm" (Canadian Institutes of Health Research, Natural Sciences and Engineering Research Council of Canada, and Social Sciences and Humanities Research Council of Canada 1998, 1.6). TPCPS 2 names as harm "anything that has a negative affect on the person's welfare" (Canadian Institutes of Health Research, Natural Sciences and Engineering Research Council of Canada, and Social Sciences and Humanities Research Council of Canada 2010, p. 22). Then, it explicitly mentions both "physical" and "psychological" harm. Special attention is likewise paid to the issue of "vulnerability." Indeed, all TCPSs have insisted that the vulnerability of the potential participant be systematically considered.

Both voluntariness and informed consent are additionally core values. TCPS 2 specifies that free and informed consent is mandatory, stating, "[c]onsent shall be given voluntarily" (3.1) and "researchers shall provide to prospective participants … full disclosure of all information necessary for making an informed decision to participate in a research project" (3.2). Among the items listed as needing to be provided is "a plain language description of all reasonably foreseeable risks" (3.2a) for it is understood that in the absence of this, the participant is in no position to make an informed decision.

Additionally, TCPS 2 lists the use of large incentives as a practice conflicting with the voluntariness of consent, stating that "incentives are … an important consideration in assessing voluntariness. Where incentives are offered to participants, they should not be so large … as to encourage reckless disregard of risks" (3.1). Correspondingly, it pointedly adds: "In considering the undue influence in research involving financial or other incentives, researchers and REBs should be sensitive to such issues as the economic circumstances of those in the pool of prospective participants and … the magnitude and probability of the harm."

The point is that the greater the likelihood and the greater the degree of harm, the less acceptable any inducement is. By the same token, what is a minor inducement for the average person could constitute a major inducement for those living in precarity. In this regard, we would add that a formula for assessing inducement commonly heard by the first author when serving on an REB is: "An incentive must not be such that it induces participants to do what they would otherwise not."

It is our conviction as researchers that all the principles and values listed here have to varying degrees been undermined by the research project in question. Opinion, however, is not the same as fact and as such, it is important that readers come *to their own conclusions*—thus, we make the quotations listed in the foregoing, as well as relevant study material, available to you.

The "Clinical" Context of ECT, the ECT Industry, and CAMH in the Industry

Electroconvulsive therapy is a procedure that consists of delivering 100–200 volts of electricity through the brain—more than sufficient to cause a grand mal seizure. Brain damage incurs both as a result of the current and of the convulsion (for details, see Breggin 2007; Burstow 2015a). Over the decades, numerous studies have proven conclusively that ECT is inherently damaging (e.g., Hartelius 1952; Calloway 1981; etc.). The largest study in history was conducted by ECT promoter Harold Sackeim (Sackeim et al. 2007). At a level far exceeding what is required for a finding of statistical significance, and with respect to every single method of delivering shock, Sackeim et al. found that standard use of ECT damages the brain and seriously impairs cognitive functioning, with the ability to remember the details of one's life particularly affected. What is likewise significant, researchers, such as Ross (2006), have established that after six weeks ECT is no more effective than placebo, which in essence means that people are being brain-damaged for nothing.

At the same time as credible studies were establishing damage and disproving effectiveness, a mammoth ECT research industry devoted to demonstrating that the "procedure" was safe and effective was moving into high gear—all overruling credible findings, all invisibilizing the everyday lives of shock survivors. Moreover, books that functioned as boss texts (e.g., Fink 1999, 2009; Abrams 2002) were spearheading a "safe and effective" narrative. By the same token, hospitals were making their reputation through ECT research. It is in this context that we must understand the ECT study.

Besides being a psychiatric teaching hospital of the U. of T., CAMH is, significantly, what activists refer to as the "shock shop of Ontario." The point is, it is to CAMH where "patients" deemed in need of ECT are routinely sent and where most Canadian ECT research occurs—itself a prestigious and lucrative adventure (for discussion of its financialization, see Andre 2009; Burstow 2015a). Indeed, it is one of the hubs in the international ECT research industry, which in turn spurs the growing use of ECT.[1]

In most institutional ethnographies, it is precisely details and contexts like these that ethnographers work on unearthing, and it is largely shedding light on such connections and the accompanying textual activations that constitutes the study. One of the facets that makes this IE activism unique is that we already understood the context—only too well. The issue was not finding out about ECT or about CAMH's place in the ECT industry. The issue was stopping this particular piece of ECT research. Toward this end, we needed to do IE-style activism to unearth and make visible the circularity, dodges, and otherwise problematic processes immediately surrounding this individual study.

OBTAINING AMMUNITION TO DRAFT THE COMPLAINT AND ITS PROCESS

All material used in the recruitment and the consent process needed to be analyzed and to accompany the complaint. Accordingly, I (Burstow) downloaded the advertisement. Other CAMH study materials collected were the flyer calling for participants and the "information and consent form"—acquired by various CAPA members, who dialed the phone number on the advertisement, presented themselves as potential participants, and requested more information.

For compilations of both the CAMH Study Material and of the Burstow /institutional correspondence, subsequently made public by a successful Freedom of Information (FOI) request and to be discussed shortly, see coalitionagainstpsychiatricassault.wordpress.com/research-paper-trails/.[2]

I additionally checked out the Craigslist category "Jobs Etcetera" to see whether there was a pattern of CAMH studies using this route to recruit participants. At that time during several months alone, there were dozens of such advertisements for different CAMH studies. A further question, accordingly, that presented itself was: Was there a systemic problem in the CAMH REB's approval or monitoring work? That noted, in the middle of August, I took the next step, for the ammunition needed to mount a complaint was now in hand.

The Complaint

On August 14 I sent an official letter of complaint to the Secretariat on Responsible Conduct of Research. Referencing all three CAMH documents, after introducing myself as a U. of T. faculty member and as someone who had sat on an REB, I detailed manifold instances where the research, in my estimation, fell short of satisfying the ethical principles and standards spelt out in the Tri-Council Policy Statement. General examples are: (a) providing monetary inducement for participants to do what they would otherwise not do (participants were being offered $645 each to agree to being electroshocked) and (b) inaccurate descriptions of the research—not only describing ECT as relatively safe but also making such misleading statements as "ECT works by telling the brain to make new brain cells" (see flyer on the Coalition Against Psychiatric Assault website).

The point here is that ECT does not "tell the brain" anything. Plus, although new brain cells do sometimes emerge via a process called "neurogenesis," they are defective cells—indeed, the result of and proof of neurological damage (see Kaplan et al. 2011), despite the positive spin commonly put on it. I concluded the letter to the Secretariat (Burstow, August 14, 2012, p. 4) as follows:

> I can indeed see ways of making this study less offensive. ... However, I see no way of making the study acceptable. While we all know that there are research situations where a degree of misleading and even downright deception would be in order, we should not be misleading participants in situations such as this. We should not be exposing participants to appreciable risk—risks to their own mental and physical integrity—in the hope of gleaning knowledge. We should not be targeting the most vulnerable for damage. We should not be bribing. We should not be preying on people's desperation and vulnerability. This piece of research does all of the foregoing. I accordingly ask the Secretariat to seriously consider ordering it stopped. Given ... the fact it has been authorized by a duly ordained body, I am likewise asking for a more general investigation into the working of the Research Ethics Board of the Centre for Addiction and Mental Health.

The gauntlet had been thrown. The target was both the study itself and the CAMH Research Ethics Board.

Change of Venue, the Next Disconnect, and the Next Stage

That the accountability process was anything but straightforward became evident in what happened next. Hours after emailing the letter, W.G. from the Secretariat called to clarify the route for complaints and to explain the institutional process. What I was guided to do was to send the letter of complaint to the "employer" of the researchers in question, after that the Secretariat would open up a file. It would be up to the employer to investigate, but the Secretariat, I was told, could take action if they felt that the complaint had not been adequately dealt with. Specifically, I was to write to the Vice President of Research at both the University of Toronto and the CAMH, with it being up to the two institutions to determine jurisdiction. I subsequently received a letter dated August 14 from the Secretariat listing exact names and addresses and reiterating that allegations of research misconduct needed to be leveled with the employer (for that route, see http://www.rcr.ethics.gc.ca/eng/policy-politique/framework-cadre/).

Already a disconnect had opened up, which raised pressing concerns about the complaints process. If the Secretariat had authority, why was it not able to directly take charge? Why was the complaint being subsumed under the category "research misconduct" when I had clearly never used such a conceptualization? And, if there is no complaint route outside that particular conceptualization, which appeared to be the case, what does that mean? What does it say about the national accountability of research when employers are the only route for objection? Is there not an inherent conflict of interest? In addition, in the long run, in situations such as this, could the Secretariat hold anyone accountable?

What added to the disconnect, albeit my complaint had, among other things, *explicitly targeted CAMH's REB*—that reality had all but disappeared. Nor was it to ever reappear except in an utterly mechanical way, despite all officials receiving a copy of the complaint. The point is, the very possibility of an objection to the *standard* workings of an REB had not been factored into the institutional processes; and as such, there was no way to investigate it. Thus, for all intents and purposes, it did not exist. That noted, I indeed did as suggested.

More Letters, More Disconnects

A flood of duly "cc'ed" letters and emails quickly ensued between several institutional operatives at CAMH, U. of T., and myself. The misconduct framework kept being reinserted despite its misfit with the complaint laid. Additionally, I was directed to the website address for the University's policy on research misconduct (http://www.sgs.utoronto.ca/Documents/Research+Misconduct+Framework.pdf). The depth of the disconnect—as well as the strategic activist pushback—can be seen in one of my responses. In this regard, I wrote:

I ... have concerns about the process for I am claiming something that is both way less serious and way more serious than what would normally be thought of as professional misconduct. As I stated in the letter, I am not claiming that the researchers broke with protocol ... or that they did not go through normal channels, or even that they promulgated what they knew to be misrepresentation, though I am clear that misrepresentation has occurred. What I am claiming is that this duly authorized piece of research fails to meet many of the Tri-Council standards by which we judge whether or not research is ethical (e.g., such principles not only as accuracy but fundamental justice, good harm/benefits ratio, not providing inducement to lead participants to agree to what they might not normally agree to). ... This lay[s] outside what is normally construed as "professional conduct" (hence my not framing it this way) but nonetheless is a reason why the research should be stopped—the ultimate purpose of the complaint. ... What I am alleging here is ... not ... personal wrong-doing. (Burstow, August 16 letter to Assistant Vice President of Research Services)

The letter ended with a reminder that time was of the essence and a request that the research be put on hold pending an investigation.

Significantly, even though I was assured that the parameters of the complaint were understood, the style and content of the emails continued to suggest otherwise. All references to problems with the CAMH's REB continued to be ignored. Plus, the statements addressed to me continued to employ the individualistic research misconduct framing—that is, "I consider allegations of *research misconduct* to be highly sensitive matters" (from Assistant Vice President August 20 email to Burstow). Nor was the suggestion that CAMH was in a conflict of interest responded to, for such possibilities too were absent from the framework. Eventually, I received a letter dated August 24 from the CEO of CAMH informing me that she had assumed responsibility for investigating the complaint.

CAMH and the Initial Victory

If an early victory of this piece of activism was the removal of the advertisement from Craigslist, a more formidable victory now ensued. On August 31, I was informed thus:

No individuals are being recruited to undergo ECT. Patients who are undergoing ECT for clinically accepted indications will have the opportunity to contribute to the knowledge of its effects. (from letter from CEO to Burstow)

In essence, what this means is that albeit the ECT study would continue, the activist IE project had successfully prevented 30 people *who would otherwise not have received ECT* from being subjected to it. Whatever else did or did not happen, as everyone in the activist community was aware, something thrilling had been achieved.What some also might consider a victory, a decision was made to convene an ad hoc panel to investigate "the complaint." As shall be seen shortly, however, what was to materialize was arguably more camouflage than inquiry.

CAMH: Its Correspondence and Processes

If one goal of the action was to reveal the face of the institution, psychiatry *as an institution* was particularly visible at this stage of the action. In quiet but significant ways, that is, at this stage of the inquiry, the institution revealed itself as utterly institution-centric. Officials appeared to have no way of understanding the world at large except as objects of their rule—otherwise known as "care." An example: In referring to the safety of the prospective research participants being recruited from outside, the CEO refers to "patient safety" (August 24 letter from CEO to Burstow) when these external down-on-their-luck individuals, whom the researchers were in essence targeting irrespective of their intention, were demonstrably not "their patients." Use of words like "patient" serve to blur the distinction between patient and participant just as the use of words like "job" blur the distinction between being a worker and being a guinea pig. It is in the putative efforts at accountability, however, that the institutional nature of CAMH's processes become most clear.

Note: At this juncture, CAMH did what it was obligated to do, given the larger structures in which it was embedded and the actions that had unfolded. It took upon itself the task of launching a major investigation, the CEO announcing:

> CAMH is taking immediate steps to investigate the allegations stated in your letter of August 14, 2012. ... We intend to have a panel of external experts review the matters that you have raised. ... We are moving forward expeditiously and will be in contact with you once the panel's work is complete. (from August 24 letter to Burstow)

On the face of it, the process was impeccable. The concerns spelled out in the complaint, it would seem—perhaps including those about CAMH's REB—were to be carefully investigated. Also, the panel was to be "external," and as such, conflict of interest appeared to have been avoided.

Look closer, however, and, you will find that even at this early stage disconnects had begun to appear. No clarification was provided of who was to be on the panel, which criteria were to be used in selecting them, or even what manner of experts these putative "experts" were. In this regard, attempting to plug one obvious possible hole, I wrote the CEO pointing out: "A critical expertise in question is expertise on what constitutes ethical research for in the absence of that, the process would be wanting" (Burstow, August 24 letter). The suggestion was never commented on—revealing in itself. Or to put this another way, "accountability" institutional-style.

Completion of the "External" Investigation: The Letter

Early the following year the panel completed its investigation and submitted its report. What is perhaps not surprising under the circumstances, except when exonerating, while detailed, the letter I received was vague; in various ways, it incorrectly depicted the nature of the complaint, and at times it appeared self-contradictory—again, a quintessential institutional account. It reads in part as follows:

> The panel did not respond to the general concerns raised in your August, 14, 2012, letter with respect to the clinical appropriateness of electroconvulsive (ECT) therapy or the investigators' compliance with the approved REB protocol. The former is a broad topic with a large body of evidence supporting the procedure … and the latter was addressed through an internal quality audit that showed full compliance. The panel confirmed that this matter does not involve a breach of research integrity or research misconduct. The study was carried out with full REB approval and the documents reviewed indicated consistent and reasonable communication between the researchers and the REB during the process of review and approval. However, the panel's recommendations focused on the need to ensure the rigor of CAMH REB processes. The panel did not find lapses in REB processes that would have compromised the integrity of the study. … We will follow each of the panel's recommendations including a review of CAMH's REB to ensure best practices for the management of issues such as recruitment, conflict of interest, and scientific review. (from CEO's January 31, 2013, letter to Burstow)

It is difficult to know what happened on this panel, including exactly what was determined. Moreover, it is impossible to know the bases for either the comparatively clear or the utterly allusive determinations—for what we have here is an institutional account—intriguing phrases wrapped up in layers of mystification. One finding, nonetheless, is crystal clear (insofar as clarity ever pertains to such accounts)—namely, that "the research does not involve a breach of research integrity or research misconduct." The finding appears to suggest that a "research misconduct" framework in some way prevailed irrespective of the nature of the complaint, which in no way alleged research misconduct, and my repeated clarification of it.

This finding, together with the decision not to query the use of ECT in any way, together with the silence that continued to enshroud the general composition of the panel, would appear to confirm our suspicions about what the panel articulated earlier. This notwithstanding, interestingly enough, one of their recommendations was precisely *a review of CAMH's REB*. Was the panel likewise uneasy about the REB's recruitment practices? In addition, what else might it have unearthed that is currently invisible to us? Short of talking with panel members, an impossibility, there was only one way to even begin to know—carefully work through the report.

Which brings us to the disheartening but expectable revelation at the end of the CEO's letter. Read the penultimate sentence and any illusion that

CAMH would willingly shed light on these questions is quickly dispelled: Writes the CEO: "The report is considered confidential." Nothing unusual about this when we consider the standard functioning of institutions—again, accountability "institutional-style." That noted, while legal issues are likely a factor here, given that what transpired is the exact opposite of transparency, and given that it is unclear why the list of recommendations itself could not be released, one cannot but wonder: What else is being hidden? By the same token, in light of what we know about CAMH per se and institutions more generally, what confidence can we have that very much, or indeed anything, will be satisfactorily addressed?

Returning to Where the Complaint Began: The Secretariat and Major Findings

With it being unclear what was happening with respect to the ECT study and with the panel appearing to vindicate it, the obvious next step was to return to the Secretariat. I accordingly called W.G. To my amazement, I discovered that the Secretariat had not only never been informed of the general "findings" of the panel but also had never been informed that its report had been submitted, or indeed its work completed—itself a disjuncture. What does it say about the foremost research oversight body when institutions can simply drop such a party from the chain of communications? That noted, the pressing question was: What would or *could* the Secretariat do?

A very formidable piece of the IE puzzle fell into place at this point. W.G. clarified the following in the phone call: Where the Secretariat is convinced that a problem still exists, more information can be requested. Moreover, where it determines that questions posed in the complaint have not been adequately addressed, it can direct the institution and researchers to attend to these. In the end additionally, if unsatisfied, it can in certain instances "pull" the study's funding. What the Secretariat cannot do (albeit an REB can) is stop the research.

In short, whatever its determinations—and in this case, to be clear, the Secretariat had not made any—this body responsible for overseeing all research in Canada could do nothing about this particular research and can do nothing about a large percentage of the research conducted under its auspices. Why? The only leverage that it has is to withdraw or threaten to withdraw funding from individual projects. Even though this may seem a formidable power, the caveat is that the Secretariat can only withdraw funding *which one of the three Councils underpinning the Secretariat themselves have provided.* Correspondingly, much of the research in Canada is either funded by other sources or unfunded. What is the implication for this particular study? Once W.G. looked up the funding details, she quickly determined that no funding came from any of the three Councils. Ergo, the Secretariat could do nothing at all.

Herein lies what is perhaps the major finding of this IE study. In the final analysis, except in very specific circumstances, the watchdog over research in

Canada in essence has "no teeth." A related finding—and we noted this very early on—is that the Secretariat has no power over the Research Ethics Boards and no mechanism by which it can even investigate a complaint against them.

But how can that be? How can it not have power over the boards the structure and very existence of which stems from specifications in the Tri-Council Policy Statement, which the Councils created and in turn authorized it to monitor? Which brings us to an even more fundamental question: In the course of this investigation, just what happened to the TCPS? It forms the basis of the complaint laid, and it is the boss text with respect to ethicality in research—that is, the text out of which all ethical research protocols in Canada are written and processed. Yet, somehow as this complaint process unfolded, it mysteriously slipped from view.

A Related IE Finding: Two Different Hierarchies and Frameworks

What underlay this mystery and what this IE activism has uncovered is that there is more than one hierarchy at work in situations involving ethical review in Canada: (1) the Tri-Council structure and (2) the structures of the universities and hospitals that house the research projects. These interact with each other in ways that disadvantage complaints. On the face of it, the Secretariat is in control of ethical review. Besides that the Secretariat has "no teeth"; what this simple depiction leaves out is that even though the REBs arise out of the Tri-Council Policy Statement, both the members of those boards and the researchers are paid employees of the university (or hospital) and ultimately accountable to them. Similarly, although the university asks faculty to sit on REBs and to make determinations in accordance with the TCPS, when it comes to complaints, the university privileges its own texts. Those texts are the universities' own research conduct and/or misconduct guidelines and the frameworks for addressing them—thus, the persistent constructing of this complaint as "research misconduct." And hence the Assistant Vice President of Research Services at the U. of T. directing "Burstow" to websites for policies related to research misconduct (www.governingcouncil.utoronto.ca/policies/ethicalr.htm and http://www.sgs.utoronto.ca/Documents/Research+Misconduct+Framework.pdf).

Although adherence to the TCPS is included in such policies (see documents on previous websites), significantly, more focal are issues like plagiarism. Correspondingly, the focus is not on research projects and their relationship to general principles but on the behavior of the individual faculty members and students. And, they primarily concern themselves with gross violation. Factoring in these texts and looking at Figure 2.2, it becomes clear what happens to the TCPS during the process:

Earlier in Figure 2.1, we saw the TCPS ensconced as the boss text, with the Tri-Council presiding over it, the Secretariat monitoring it, the REBs in the middle, and the research projects at the bottom. Once a general complaint about a study is lodged, however, a very different hierarchy appears.

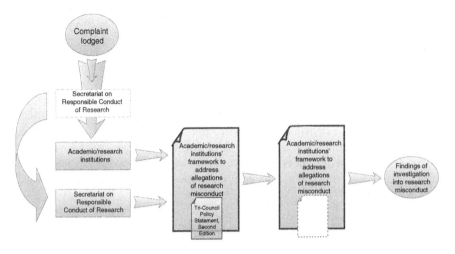

Figure 2.2   The textual and hierarchical disconnects

The presumptive boss text is still there, but it is no longer centered. As shown in the lower part of Figure 2.2, the Secretariat is still concerned with the TCPS; however, even by their own understanding, it is now only part of a larger framework—one over which the Secretariat has negligible control. When it comes to the academic bodies that take authority over the complaint (see top sequence), similarly, the TCPS has all but disappeared (see "ghost" version of the TCPS on the right side of the diagram)!

A complaint that a piece of research falls significantly short of satisfying the ethical principles articulated in the TCPS herein translates into an inquiry into blatant violations of university conduct guidelines by employees. In the process, instead of a firm check on pieces of research transpiring, a route has been established whereby problematic protocols can actually be reaffirmed. Of course, the Secretariat can always reassert the significance of the TCPS and draw the researchers and the university back to the questions posed in complaints. As already noted, however, the Secretariat has "no teeth."

Short of major changes ensuing, irrespective of intentions, herein lies a profound limitation on research accountability in Canada.

SUMMARIZING, ANALYZING, REFLECTING, AND RECOMMENDING

We began this chapter with a colossal disjuncture. ECT survivors and their allies woke one morning to an advertisement on Craigslist that was, it has been argued, distressingly misleading. It offered a sum of money significant enough that it was reasonably foreseeable that it would induce those down on their luck to do what they otherwise were highly unlikely to—sign up for an ECT study, thereby placing themselves at risk of sustaining prolonged cognitive dysfunction and damage. This chapter has traced the twists and turns of the activism that almost instantly ensued, showing how it fed the IE analysis and vice versa. Successes of the activism as they have materialized include: getting the advertisement removed, stopping the public recruitment, and forcing an investigation.

What the activism revealed about the operations of the CAMH is that its researchers frequently use recruitment processes that appear to fall short of TCPS standards (e.g., see section quoted earlier on the nullifying of voluntariness through unfair inducement); that CAMH's REB was not preventing such processes; and that, to varying degrees, circularity and mystification characterize CAMH's attempts at accountability. If this is worrisome, it is not surprising. The big surprise is what was unearthed about research oversight in Canada—namely, despite a mammoth bureaucracy and despite the existence of a body that ostensibly oversees research, that body has very little power to stop unethical research.

Indeed, once a general complaint is lodged, except in cases where one of the three Councils "controls the purse strings," both the Secretariat and the actual ethical principles established for research in Canada become peripheral at best. Related findings include: It is the employer who looks into and acts on complaints. Invisibilization, mystification, and various degrees of conflict of interest are endemic to the oversight process. There are two hierarchies, and the workers in each activate very different texts. Similarly, once a general complaint has been lodged, the focus is on the individual researcher as opposed to the study.

If this is bad news about the state of research oversight in Canada generally, we would point out, it is particularly bad for communities such as the one experiencing the disjuncture. The point is, what would look like serious skirting of the TCPS principles to an "outsider" would look like business as usual to members of the psychiatric regime. Moreover, a very high percentage of psychiatric research is funded by multinational pharmaceutical companies and other manufacturers of "clinical substances" (see Whitaker 2010)—in other words, *not by the Tri-Council*. Ergo, the Secretariat has no leverage and what follows, no way to stop research or to enforce changes. What exactly does this mean?

In essence, that unless the REB is rigorous, the very researchers who are most likely to place people in physical jeopardy, moreover, who are attracting particularly vulnerable participants (e.g., researchers whose studies involve major psychiatric interventions) can entice and mystify with relative impunity. A frightening implication.

Recommendations specific to psychiatric research are beyond the scope of this chapter. The following are suggestions for changes to research oversight more generally—and these clearly arise from the IE activism:

1. The processes need to be clearer and more transparent.
2. Where a substantive complaint is involved, the study itself should be assessed.
3. The TCPS should be used when investigating complaints.
4. Authority for investigating complaints needs to be vested in independent organizations that minimally are not the employer and do not start or stop with the employer.

5. Either the Secretariat or some other independent body should have the authority to put a halt to pieces of research or to mandate changes.
6. A route for complaints against an REB needs to be established.

To be clear, not that either of us believes that genuine accountability is possible when it comes to a ruling regime as plagued by credibility problems as psychiatry has been shown to have (for details, see Whitaker and Cosgrove 2015; Burstow 2015a). And, not that either of us are unaware that consolidating the power of national authorities could mean little more than further ruling from on high, with antioppression research especially negatively impacted—although for the most part, the travesty that psychiatry perpetrates in the name of research continues to be justifiable. As such, these recommendations are hardly being put forward as ultimate answers.

That noted, we have strayed a long way from the initial disjuncture and the community that mobilized around it. So, it is with this community that we end this chapter.

The Survivors and the Activists: The Story Continues

As the action unfolded, there were a number of high spots for survivors and activists. The most thrilling of these was when recruitment from the general population stopped—a genuine victory. At the same time, no one was under the illusion that anything either permanent or fundamental had been achieved. The reality is: The study continued, and recruitment of a similar nature could start up at any time. Correspondingly, on any given day, CAMH workers associated with what are minimally worrisome studies were going about their duties—returning phone calls, placing advertisements, assuring participants that the procedure was safe, turning on the EEG machine. In other words, it was life as usual at the "Shock Shop of Ontario." This understood, once CAMH's investigation into the study was finished, a new stage of activism ensued. If the primary goal of the first stage had been "stopping CAMH," the primary goal of the second activism stage was using the study and the investigation to do the very thing that its carefully preserved secrecy was intended to prevent—expose CAMH.

On the face of it, this was not easy—again, for institutional reasons. Only Burstow had a copy of the relevant correspondence, and given that she was a U. of T. employee, releasing it was somewhat hazardous. The solution was a Freedom of Information request. Thus, in early 2013 a CAPA member (J.W.) filed a request with CAMH's FOI officer; and indeed in the fullness of time, the complete correspondence was released. CAPA then placed the correspondence (minus items labeled confidential) on its website where they function as a research trail—a major act of exposure in its own right. These documents having been made public; correspondingly, with the use of them, the authors proceeded to construct the chapter that you are currently reading—a further act of exposure and resistance.

Additionally, Burstow (2015b) published an article in the *Journal of Humanistic Psychology* that has been widely read by "mental health professionals." It makes visible not only what happened at CAMH but also employs the correspondence to establish what was done; but mostly she writes about what psychiatric researchers routinely do. In the process, recruitment processes and standards employed in psychiatric clinical trials are questioned more generally.

That noted, the activists have not finished their work for the disjuncture persists—the particular juncture involving CAMH, the larger disjuncture vis-á-vis what psychiatric researchers can do and *routinely* do—and indeed, with impunity. What new initiatives will the various activists pursue? Also, in light of the newly acquired penchant for IE analysis, which other pieces of the IE puzzle might fall into place in the process? Intriguing questions but impossible to answer—for both figuratively and literally, that chapter has yet to be written. In other words, in the parlance of the media, "stay tuned."

NOTES

1. ECT, significantly, has been dramatically on the rise worldwide. See, in this regard, Wells and Ziomislic (2012).
2. For legal reasons, all correspondence marked "confidential" have been excluded.

REFERENCES

Abrams, R. (2002). *Electroconvulsive therapy* (4th. ed.). New York: Oxford University Press.

Andre, L. (2009). *Doctors of deception*. New Brunswick: Rutgers University Press.

Breggin, P. (2007). ECT damages the brain: Disturbing news for patients and shock doctors alike. *Ethical Human Psychology and Psychiatry, 9*, 83 ff.

Burstow, B. (2015a). *Psychiatry and the business of madness*. New York: Palgrave Macmillan.

Burstow, B. (2015b). Recruitment for psychiatric treatment trials: An ethical investigation. *Journal of Humanistic Psychology*. doi: 101177/0022167815594546. First published on July 5, 2015.

Calloway, S. (1981). ECT and cerebral atrophy. *Acta Psychiatrica Scandinavica, 64*, 441–445.

Canadian Institutes of Health Research, Natural Sciences and Engineering Research Council of Canada, and Social Sciences and Humanities Research Council of Canada. (1998). *Tri-Council Policy Statement: Ethical conduct for research involving humans*.

Canadian Institutes of Health Research, Natural Sciences and Engineering Research Council of Canada, and Social Sciences and Humanities Research Council of Canada. (2010). *Tri-Council Policy Statement: Ethical conduct for research involving humans*, December.

Fink, M. (1978). Efficacy and safety of induced seizures (EST) in man. *Comprehensive Psychiatry, 19*, 1–18.

Fink, M. (1999). *Electroshock: Restoring the mind*. New York: Oxford University Press.

Fink, M. (2009). *Electroconvulsive therapy: A guide for practitioners and their patients*. New York: Oxford University Press.

Hartelius, H. (1952). Cerebral changes following electrically induced convulsions. *Acta Psychiatr Neurol Scand, 28*(supplement), 1–128.

Inquiry into Psychiatry. (2005). *Transcripts of testimony.* Retrieved on November 4, 2012 from http://coalitionagainstpsychiatricassault.wordpress.com/articles/personal-narratives/

Kaplan, G., Vasterling, J., & Vedak, C. (2011). *Braind-derived neurotropic factor in traumatic brain injury, post-traumatic stress disorder, and their co-morbid conditions.* Retrieved on April 12, 2016 from http://www.ectresources.org/ECTscience/Kaplan__G___et_al__2010__BDNF_caused_by_trauma__brain_damage.pdf

Phoenix Rising Collective. (Ed.) (1984). Testimony on electroshock. *Phoenix Rising, 3 and 4*, 16A–22A.

Ross, C. (2006). The sham ECT literature: Implications for consent to ECT. *Ethical Human Psychology and Psychiatry, 8*, 17–28.

Sackeim, H., Prudic, J., Fuller, R., et al. (2007). The cognitive effects of electroconvulsive therapy in community settings. *Neuropsychopharmacology, 32*, 244–255.

Smith, G. (1990). Political activist as ethnographer. *Social Problems, 37*, 629–648.

Wells, J., & Ziomislic, D. (2012). *Experts weigh in on the alarming rise in use of electroconvulsive therapy.* Retrieved December 13, 2013 from http://www.thestar.com/news/canada/2012/12/23/experts_weigh_in_on_alarming_rise_in_use_of_electroconvulsive_therapy.html.

Whitaker, R. (2010). *Anatomy of an epidemic.* New York: Broadway Paperbacks.

Whitaker, R., & Cosgrove, L. (2015). *Psychiatry under the influence.* New York: Palgrave Macmillan.

CHAPTER 3

A Kind of Collective Freezing-Out: How Helping Professionals' Regulatory Bodies Create "Incompetence" and Increase Distress

Chris Chapman, Joanne Azevedo, Rebecca Ballen, and Jennifer Poole

INTRODUCING OURSELVES, OUR PROJECT, AND OUR PROBLEMATIC

We are four social work researchers.[1] Although diverse in terms of psychiatric involvement and self-identification as *Mad*, antipsychiatric activists, consumer-survivors, and so on, we have all had experiences deemed abnormal and pathological by psychiatry. We share the political dream of a world in which such experiences are held and known very differently.

Unequivocally, we believe that the various diverse experiences banded together as "mental illness" within psychiatry have nothing at all to do with "competence" in the helping professions. At all, at all. Besides indeed, this is the crux of the story that we hope to tell. That is, the equation of presumptive "mental illness" with "incompetence" is precisely the problematic that we hope to illuminate.

Now without a doubt, there are many reasons why a person may not be a good helping professional. Some people are not very warm; do not take their responsibilities to others seriously; are terrible listeners; always think they know best; or do explicit and egregious racist, sexist, transphobic, and otherwise

C. Chapman (✉) • J. Azevedo • R. Ballen
School of Social Work, York University, Toronto, ON, Canada
e-mail: chap@yorku.ca

J. Poole
School of Social Work, Ryerson University, Toronto, ON, Canada
e-mail: jpoole@ryerson.ca

© The Editor(s) (if applicable) and The Author(s) 2016
B. Burstow (ed.), *Psychiatry Interrogated*,
DOI 10.1007/978-3-319-41174-3_3

41

oppressive things. Many qualities might make someone a less than supportive helping professional; having been labeled with a psychiatric diagnosis is not among those things. And our research strongly supports this stance.

Neither the human experiences pathologized as "mental illness" nor the labels attached to them prevent a person from excelling in the helping professions. Still, the very fact of a practitioner's psychiatric diagnosis, from whatever point in her life, activated through assumptions of "incompetence," disseminated among the wrong colleagues, and reported to her regulatory body can utterly destroy an otherwise successful career and can leave one's life "in shambles." That is the story of this chapter. It is not the story of "professional incompetence" because of "mental illness." It is the story of helping professionals actively constructing other professionals as "incompetent" because of utterly normative sanism/mentalism (Birnbaum 1960; Chamberlin 1990; Perlin 1992), and its moral and political differentiations of who is and is not a valuable and competent human (Chapman 2013; Poole et al. 2012; Poole and Ward 2013; Reid and Poole 2013).

The research underpinning this chapter includes interviews and document analysis, guided by institutional ethnography (IE). In it per se, we discuss interviews we have conducted with two nurses who lost the right to practice. For each, the initial questioning of their "competence," following years of previously living lives in which they had psychiatric diagnoses and also worked as professionals, constituted a profound disjuncture. The subsequent verdict—"unfit to practice"—was all the more so. Neither one had any way to make sense of how or why this was happening. As a result, they did not initially understand how serious it was; neither could have foreseen a future in which they would never be allowed to practice again. The calling into question of their "competence," in both cases, seemed to come "out of the blue" and both seem to have originated not with their diagnosis or any particularly acute period of difficulty, but rather with mentioning the diagnosis to the wrong person.

This disjuncture—this situated "what on earth is happening to me?"—provides an entry point for the interrogation of the system of professional regulation of who is and is not "fit to practice." In our home province, regulatory bodies that do this work include the College of Nurses of Ontario (CNO), the Ontario College of Social Workers and Social Service Workers (OCSWSSW), and the newly minted College of Registered Psychotherapists and Mental Health Therapists of Ontario. It is telling that this new College just sprang up because systems of professionalization and regulation continue to gain headway. As another example of this, Social Work, which has been regulated by OCSWSSW since 2000, is now threatened with a new national body attempting to take it upon itself to introduce standardized competency exams for Social Work graduates (Canadian Council of Social Work Regulators 2013).

With the old and predictable story that they exist to protect the public, this would work against diversity and innovation in Social Work education and would depoliticize the study of Social Work as a site of both everyday structural violence and potential radical social transformation. (For a sense of the diversity of perspectives on competencies, see Aronson and Hemingway 2011; Birnbaum and Silver 2011; Campbell 2011; Carignan 2011; Fook 2011; Bogo et al. 2011; Rossiter and Heron 2011; Todd 2011).

Professionalization and professional regulation has served to delegitimize alternative helping practitioners for centuries. In seventeenth century England, the College of Physicians "was granted permission to fine unlicensed practitioners" (Burstow 2015, p. 32). This was a significant step in a lengthier process starting with Medieval witch-hunts, so "bit by bit women practitioners were pushed out" of the work of getting paid to help in Europe by the 1800s (2015, p. 38). This started with doctors' denunciations of the Church's understanding of witches—countering that these unfairly persecuted women were actually mad (therefore more appropriately under medical jurisdiction than that of the Church). Many of these women were healers responsible for community practices such as performing abortions and administering herbal remedies. The medical challenge to witch-hunts was thus at once a challenge to the moral authority of the Church and of the women health practitioners, who were thereby rendered "incompetent" (2015, pp. 30–31).

Jurisdictional claims to this or that moral and political sphere of life always have been interlocked with other differentiations of worthy from unworthy humans—sexism as in the aforementioned example; nonetheless, this is inseparably a history of racism and colonialism, if we consider that these European misogynist jurisdictional claims were eventually imposed on every corner of the world through European imperialism, colonialism, and neocolonialism (Mills 2014). Again inseparably, European imperialism has likewise devastated local practices in which those who transgressed binary gender differentiations were long respected as healers—that is, the two-spirit people in Indigenous communities in what is now called Canada, the US, and the hijra communities in South Asia (Alaers 2010).

The regulation of who is and is not "fit" to practice as a helping professional connects to a wider problematic or field of political, ethical, and scholarly concern. That problematic is this: Although framed as apolitical scientific phenomena, in everyday life psychiatric diagnoses morally and politically disqualify people from being imaginable as "competent" human beings. Countless systems are implicated in this extra-local problematic, including many systems peopled by helping professionals. As part of its duty to serve and to protect the public interest, regulatory bodies, such as the OCSWSSW and the CNO, claim they are required to have a formal Fitness to Practice process. Part III of the 1998 Social Work and Social Service Act (SWSSA) states:

[The] Fitness to Practice Committee will hold a hearing to determine any allegation of incapacity on the part of a member of the College. The Fitness to Practice Committee may, after a hearing, find a member of the College to be incapacitated if, in its opinion, the member is suffering from a physical or mental condition or disorder such that the member is unfit to continue to carry out his or her professional responsibilities.

Similarly, the CNO states: "The Fitness to Practice Committee determines whether a nurse is incapacitated and suffering from a physical or mental condition or disorder that is affecting, *or could affect*, her or his practice." (emphasis added). Both Colleges, then, specifically name "mental condition or disorder" as a possible cause of unfitness. As such, the Colleges position themselves as guardians of public safety and position individual (i.e., psychiatrized) professionals as potentially "incapacitated" and dangerous.

When helping professionals are found unfit, consequences may include revoking or suspending their certificate of registration or adding conditions. How do we unhook the helping professions from psychiatry, from this punitive medical model of disability, and from our own practices of scrutinizing and punishing in the name of public safety?

Although the study began with "through the grapevine" reports of social workers having lost the right to practice, the participants discussed in this chapter are both nurses. Their stories are very similar to what we have heard informally about the OCSWSSW, and we suspect that this process is not limited to these two professions.

JANET'S STORY

Our first entry point into this situation is by way of an accomplished, scholarly, and popular nurse who had been practicing for more than 20 years. Her name is Janet, she is English-speaking, and she identifies as white. After casually sharing her decades-long history of "depression" with a new manager, Janet was placed under intense scrutiny and surveillance, and subsequently reported to the CNO. The College found her incapable of practicing, and so she is now no longer allowed to work. She has been forever changed by this ruling; she lives a devalued life, in poverty and cut off from the profession she served so long and loves. What began as an unremarkable conversation between colleagues has, in her words, come close to ending her life.

In an interview with her, the first in our inquiry, the sequence of events becomes clear (see Figure 3.1 in section "Discussion"). After qualifying as a nurse in Ontario, Janet worked for 20 years without incident. Promoted and well-thought-of, Janet rose in the ranks at her "supportive" hospital, had a spotless record, and began graduate studies. She was an expert trainer and ward nurse and also was involved in both research and policy development. Throughout this time, she experienced feelings attributed to "depression" and substance use, related to a history of family "trauma" and grief. She actively sought and received support as needed, "was never hospitalized," and overall can be said to have clearly excelled in her life and career. In 2007, the hospital where she was based for all her years of work was amalgamated with another.

It is at this moment that things start to shift. Janet's role changes to more of a "desk job," her coworkers changed, and she was assigned a new manager called "Jerry." Given her two decades of diverse experience, spotless record, and graduate studies, Janet wonders today if Jerry felt that she was after her

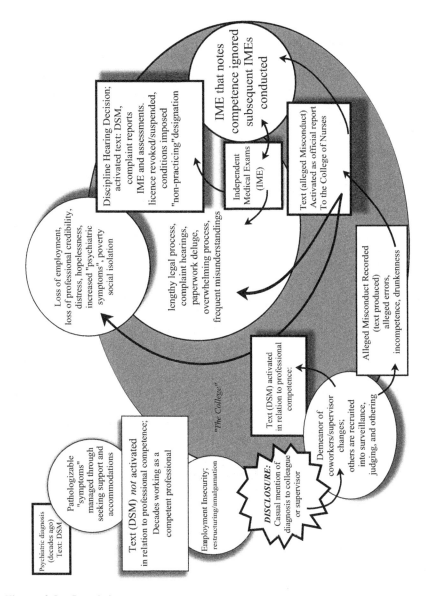

Figure 3.1 Janet's journey

job. In casual conversation and wishing for Jerry to know her better as a person (and thus for Janet to feel more secure in this new workplace), Janet shares her history with Jerry, disclosing her depression and membership in a 12-step group. Janet asks Jerry not to tell anyone. Jerry's demeanor changes immediately. "It was a 180," says Janet. Jerry subsequently enlists Janet's coworkers to "watch her" and speaks to patients about her too. Jerry begins to compile a file of notes, some of which claim Janet is "drunk" on the job, that she is frequently absent, and that she is incapable of looking after patients.

As a result of this harassment and surveillance, Janet begins to feel "very uncomfortable" at the hospital. To manage the distress stemming from the scrutiny and denigration, she reenrolls in a 12-step group, completes a residential substance use treatment program, and asks for an accommodation to shorten her shifts. Then, "out of the blue" in 2010, she receives a copy of a formal eight-page complaint about her made to the CNO. This text questions her capacity, "knowledge and skills," and sanity. It includes the aforementioned and anonymized notes on her performance.

From this point on, she is no longer allowed to practice as a nurse. She is directed to have an Independent Medical Exam (IME) with a psychiatrist of the College's choosing. When this exam concludes that she is functioning above average and should be allowed to work, the College orders her to see another psychiatrist, and then another and another over the next few years—all the while not allowing her to work. Of the psychiatrists who questioned her capacity, Janet describes utterly arbitrary facts being used against her. One College-approved psychiatrist suggests that she may be "bi-polar" because she changed her hair color. Another is concerned about the amount of eye make-up she wears to her appointment. Eventually, Janet is ordered to have another full IME; the report about it, like the first, evaluates her as "above average," stating that there are no concerns with her "mental health." During this entire process, she has no income.

There is no investigation into Jerry's harassment of Janet, and Jerry subsequently leaves the hospital. The College's process continues. Janet's own psychologist is not allowed to attest to her abilities. The CNO decides to hold a five-day hearing. Janet does not feel strong enough to attend the hearing because of the toll this process has had on her, so in her absence the College decides to make her a non-practicing nurse. Janet appeals the decision, working with her own lawyer and lodging multiple grievances. Now eight years into this complaint process, Janet is considering taking her case to the Ontario Human Rights Tribunal; however, her lawyer "is trying to talk her out of it," and she has been "told she will lose the case." Janet has depleted all of her financial resources on this process and is without much emotional support. She wants to be a part of a class action lawsuit against the College.

We can trace the presence of certain texts in this sequence of events. First, there is the set of notes compiled about Janet by her manager and coworkers. Second, these notes are folded into the official complaint. Next comes the IME, to which Janet is subjected twice. These texts hold a particularly important place in the process because they demonstrate the dominance of psychiatry in the complaint process and the power of psychiatric terms, practices, and decisions. Yet another text is the "decision" or ruling—a text that comes after countless others are produced and reviewed as part of the hearing. Finally, there are the texts still circulating, such as those being filed with the Ontario Human Rights Tribunal and being readied for what Janet hopes will be a class action lawsuit. Additionally, in Janet's possession are countless articles, reports, letters, emails, and notes saved over the last eight years, all of which attest to her suffering.

IKMA'S STORY

Our second interviewee, Ikma, is an intelligent, wise, and passionate woman who obtained her nursing degree in the last decade (see Figure 3.2 later). Ikma identifies as a racialized woman from Africa and as a survivor of war. She has worked throughout her nursing studies as a Personal Support Worker (PSW) with an agency that provides contract staff to hospitals and other nursing facilities. She was diagnosed with "bi-polar disorder" prior to becoming licensed as a nurse. Like Janet, Ikma worked successfully as a nurse for years before being deemed "unfit" to practice, and the complaint against her was brought only after she made a casual disclosure to someone at her workplace.

Ikma was unable to find permanent work after completing her nursing degree so she was forced to accept temporary contract jobs. As a precarious worker, she experienced frequent job changes that forced her to spend significant resources traveling to/from work all over southern Ontario. This left her feeling very disconnected and displaced, but she attended to her own welfare by being selective about her shifts and not working nights. Thus, she fared well for several years in spite of the precarity. One day, however, she shared with a colleague that she had been previously diagnosed as "bi-polar." She was immediately threatened with being reported to the CNO. She started to feel unwelcome and unsafe at her workplace. She became the subject of gossip within her professional community, and no longer felt like part of the team. There were moments in which she felt "set up"—as if her colleagues were trying to get her into trouble.

Ikma's life took an abrupt turn one day a few years ago when she was late for work at a site at which she had never previously worked. She called ahead to advise her employer that she would be late because of bad traffic caused by an Afro-Caribbean street festival. Her employer misunderstood the situation and interpreted this to mean that Ikma was late because of having partied at this festival all night. Her arrival at work was further delayed when she could not find the unit to which she had been assigned. As had happened so often in the past, Ikma's assignment was in a new, unfamiliar hospital. She wandered around trying to find the unit, eventually gave up and phoned her agency to get directions, and ultimately located the correct unit.

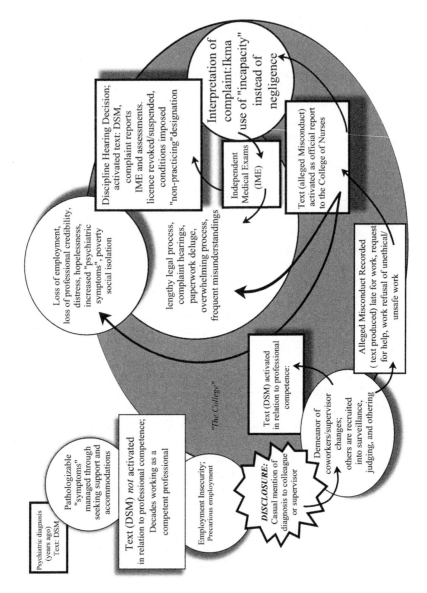

Figure 3.2   Ikma's journey

Upon arriving, Ikma was assigned a heavy workload, with many patients who had very complex medical needs. One was particularly difficult, behaving in a manner that was verbally abusive and threatening. When Ikma asked for help, however, her coworkers ignored her. Later that same day, she was asked to conduct a routine nursing procedure that had a clear protocol requiring two nurses, very specific documentation, and two signatures. Again none of her colleagues were willing work with her on the task. Instead, contrary to protocol, she was advised to do it alone. Ikma understood this to be a significant breach in protocol and was concerned that she was being "set up." Feeling overwhelmed, without support, and unable to work safely and ethically on the unit, Ikma decided to leave.

A few days later, Ikma received a termination letter. She had lost her job with the placement agency. She subsequently received a letter from the CNO outlining that she had been reported to them. Initially, she was accused of abandoning a patient, but a subsequent letter stated that she was retroactively designated as "incapacitated" because of "mental illness." She lost her license to practice as a nurse and any hope of regaining it in the future would have to be determined by a CNO-designated psychiatrist.

As an immediate result, Ikma experienced a sharp decline in her health and soon underwent her first of many in-patient hospitalizations; this had never happened previous to the CNO complaint. She describes having been deluged with documents from the College that she did not understand. She participated in a psychiatric assessment as requested by the College and was asked to sign a consent form allowing the CNO to examine her medical records, including those that predated her certification with the College. She says: "I made another issue for myself by signing a consent form. I thought if I signed the consent, the College could see that I was doing well in the hospital and I could get my licence and everything would go away." She believed that the information would support her defense and her return to work. Instead, she says it just opened up more issues, allowed the College to contact her former employers, and created a lot of discrepancies in her record. As she notes, "they don't have their story right."

Sometime after her dismissal from her nursing position, while hospitalized for "depression," there was a period when Ikma was struggling to eat. Her parents were cited in the hospital chart as believing that she wanted to die. Based on her parents' comments, Ikma was designated a "danger to herself or others." This provided the necessary rationale for further consultations with her family members without her consent. They mused about her use of marijuana, and this was then taken as "evidence" of possible drug abuse. She was also "re-diagnosed" with "bi-polar disorder" and "depressive" episodes. Although Ikma does not dispute she has "mental health" issues, she disagrees with the diagnosis of bi-polar.

Throughout this progression, Ikma did not understand the Fitness to Practice assessment process and did not realize, for example, that she was expected to attend the hearings. She believed that her participation in the psychiatric assessment was all that was required. But because she missed her hearing, she was deemed to have been "in breach," so her license was revoked. Over a year later, she was directed to attend another hearing. This time she missed the hearing because she did not receive the notice because she was in the hospital. This nevertheless was considered another "breach."

Almost 40 months after the initial complaint, Ikma has ceased all communication with the College and sought her own legal counsel. Her lawyer has advised her not to fight the designation of "incapacitated" because he thinks she has a better chance of getting her license back if she accepts the designation and then complies with the College's directives related to "mental health treatment." The College has continued to monitor her activities, insisting on getting information about where she is working—regardless of the fact that she is not currently employed in a medical setting. Ikma was advised that she must report wherever she is working so that they can verify she is abiding by the restriction to not work as a nurse. She has been directed to attend counseling, but she cannot afford to pay for it. Ikma therefore is volunteering in a community center as a way to gain access to the counseling that she cannot afford.

Discussion

Janet and Ikma faced particular kinds of harassment and institutional disqualification, but both of their experiences appear to have followed a similar sequence of events. The sequence of each's events is illustrated in Figures 3.1 and 3.2, respectively.

First, both workers had been diagnosed *previously* but had fared very well in their lives following these diagnoses. That is not to say that they did not ever experience difficulties related to the experiences underlying the diagnoses, but they were able to manage their own distress effectively through peer and professional support, selectivity around working hours, and so on. Both then experienced challenging work conditions (amalgamation and reassignment with Janet; precarious casual employment with Ikma). As a result of these unfavorable working conditions, each experienced a lack of professional and institutional support. Both made informal disclosures to coworkers about their diagnoses and, in response, both experienced very negative immediate reactions and began to be harassed on the job—Janet through increased surveillance from colleagues and patients who her supervisor recruited to keep tabs on her, and Ikma through a threat to report her to the College.

In both cases, this was followed by formal complaints made to the CNO; a confusing, long-lasting and exhaustive legal process during which both experienced multiple psychiatric assessments and intrusions as dictated by the College. Ultimately, each had their licenses to practice revoked, which resulted in a loss of income and a significant increase in distress, resulting in poverty and more pathologizable "symptoms." In spite of all that, both still want to work, love their profession, and are seeking a means of reinstatement through independent legal advice.

These women do not know each other. They come from entirely different locations and yet what has happened to them demonstrates the contention "of IE that ruling happens through ... the activation of texts" (Burstow 2015, p. 18). Both are "ruled" by the power of psychiatric regulation and discipline, which continues to destroy many lives. During her interview, Janet noted, "I had never experienced stigma and discrimination before this," but that now she well understands "there is absolutely no support" for people "like her." Speaking to ruling texts, she asks: "If I had breast cancer, would they be doing IMEs on me? No." If given a chance she would say to the College, "What's it going to take? You'll have no nurses if you keep this up." She adds, "I think I am fit to practice ... and it wasn't just me who thought I was good at it. All of my experience makes me better qualified to deal with any form of stigma and discrimination but especially mental health. I have understood it and experienced it."

How is it, we ask, that two very different nurses with dissimilar diagnoses, ages, employment histories, positioning relative to race and racism, and so on were put through such a strikingly similar process? Also what can the discrepancies or particularities teach us about institutional power, professional regulation, and psychiatrization?

Selective Activation of Texts and Selective Constitution of Agency

According to Dorothy Smith, tracing the activation of texts is essential to institutional ethnography because texts "create a juncture between the local and specific ... and the extra-local and abstract" (Widerberg 2004, p. 180). Texts connect the local workings of power with systemic or structural violence and inequity and the extra-local discourses that rationalize the violence toward them. In the stories of Ikma and Janet, this is clear in the ways that colleagues' unfavorable observations of them are put together into a formal complaint with the CNO. These complaints become organized through institutional structures and procedures and are interpreted through "sanist" discourse into an account of Ikma and Janet as "mentally ill" and *therefore* as potentially "unfit to practice."

Significantly, we do not know whether Ikma's colleagues knew of her psychiatric diagnosis before the fateful day that began with getting stuck in traffic and finding a new hospital difficult to navigate—two very common experiences that do not ordinarily lend themselves to a person being deemed "mentally ill" or "incompetent." It could be the case in fact that Ikma's colleagues may have initially mistreated her and judged her based on prejudices associated with what Benjamin (2003) has named anti-Black racism rather than sanism. Indeed, initially she was let go because of a specific behavioral infraction, however unfairly and out of context, that was not initially connected to psychiatrization either by her employer or the College. But, as this moved through the procedures at the extra-local level of the CNO, it was joined with other colleagues' concerns stemming only from her psychiatric diagnosis.

Only then did the behavioral infraction become evidence that Ikma was too "mentally ill" to be a nurse. It quite possibly had nothing to do with sanism at its most local occurrence, but then came to have everything to do with it once "mental illness" became available to someone at some point as an explanation for her behavior. This obscuring of racism into normalized and seemingly race-neutral pathologization, we would add, is a common way that racism and sanism, or disablism, interlock (Callow 2013; Chapman 2013). Indeed, Abdillahi et al. have named this interlocking anti-Black sanism (in press).

Additionally, nothing Ikma or Janet did would necessarily lead one to interpret their actions as having anything to do with either mental illness or incompetence—the two are conflated in the problematic we are exploring. Smith notes that if you explore how "texts enter into the organizing of any corporation ... a person can be regarded separated from her tasks, that is as something different and/or more than her activities" (cited in Widerberg 2004, p. 181). The texts that Ikma's and Janet's colleagues generated about them constitute inaccurate representations. However, the texts get taken up—by their respective employers first, and then by the College—as evidence of what kind of practitioners they are, what kind of persons they are, really. Burstow describes this as "the work of transforming them into creatures of the system" (2015, p. 115).

Ikma and Janet become creatures of the system, of course. Their colleagues also become creatures of the system through the process of being directed by their supervisor to carefully observe and document concerns. We know that this took place in Janet's story, and we can anticipate that: first, Ikma's colleagues' supervisor would have asked them to account for what happened on the day they drove her away; and second, that they would have had a vested interest in describing what took place in a way that did not position themselves as having driven her away.

Whatever form these documented concerns initially took—an official Critical Incident Report, something scribbled on the back of a napkin, or something else (i.e., the doing of the documentation) made them a participant in the sanist problematic we are exploring. They were called on to be agents of the regulation of who is and is not fit to practice, and they took this task on as a part of their nursing duties. After all, helping professionals are exceptionally good at documenting these kinds of observations about people deemed ill and/or incompetent through case notes, patient charts, and so forth. It is just that this does not normally extend to fellow helping professionals.

Smith encourages us to consider that "not only subjects are constituted; so is agency ... [and that] 'agency' must be seen as constituted in the authorized texts of organization" (Smith 2001, p. 185). The capacity to make things happen is not naturally connected to what one does or to how well one does it. It may well be the case that Ikma or Janet were each the most "competent" nurse working at a given time when an unfavorable observation was made of her, but they were not granted the agency or capacity to judge others' "competence."

In Ikma's story, we certainly can imagine she could have made a compelling case against her colleagues who did not assist her with the abusive patient and directed her to break protocol. But our opinion is not that she was more "competent" than them—we are in no position to judge that. The point is that these colleagues were only in the position that they were because the extra-local organization of their relations made it so. As Smith (2001) writes, "agents are constituted in organizational/institutional discourse. Whatever the actual work of those involved ... agency is recognized ... in terms of organizational/institutional status ... [so that] people's work in a given setting is co-ordinated to accomplish organizational or institutional objectives" (pp. 186–187). These objectives may not be known or acknowledged by those who are enlisted as their agents.

So, again, Ikma's coworkers that day may have had no idea that they would be contributing to the loss of her registration because of "mental illness." They may not have interpreted or known her as mentally ill at all. Yet, their capacity to play a key role in her delegitimization was enabled by the organizational structure, procedures, and discourses of the College.

The corollary of this is that in these two stories we also find texts that were *not* activated and people who were *not granted agency* because the ruling structures, procedures, and discourses did not permit it. Ikma's potential to lodge a complaint against her coworkers that day is one example. Janet's grievances against her supervisor, Jerry, are another. What we might imagine as a key difference between Janet's grievances and Ikma's potential complaint is that Janet actually filed them—but this difference, as it were, made no difference. Janet filed texts that grieved Jerry's harassment. But these grievances, these particular texts, were not activated. Janet was not granted agency through the discourse of the College. As cited, Janet stated to us, "I think I am fit to practice ... and it wasn't just me who thought I was good at it."

We can imagine that she said something like that to the CNO at some point, and also to Jerry. We can imagine too that some of her colleagues may also have reported accounts of Janet's "competence" to Jerry and/or the College. Nevertheless, accounts of her competence were not activated by the structures and discourses governing what happened. Consequently, Janet's requests for her shifts to be reduced because of the harassment she was experiencing were denied. Within the process of her delegitimization, this could not be understood as an attempt to take care of herself in an impossible situation caused by workplace harassment; it could only be taken up as further evidence of her "ineptitude" because it was stories and framings of her ineptitude that were exclusively granted agency.

If this seems like an extreme position that we are taking, consider this: Janet had two College-designated psychiatrists find her "competent" to practice through the IMEs the College required her to undergo. But the texts that documented those particular psychiatric assessments were not activated. Those psychiatrists were somehow not granted agency to determine the outcome of the hearing. Instead, musings about her hair and makeup (from two other psychiatrists) were activated and entered into the official record. So it would seem that it is not only a matter of official categories (e.g., nurse versus psychiatrist) that might serve as an official explanation of why Janet's own psychologist could not testify about her "competence." Rather, various people inhabiting the same institutional category (i.e., CNO-appointed psychiatrists) were granted unequal agency. In addition, this was based on, it seems, their stance vis-à-vis Janet's sanity and competence.

When Texts Are Not Present

Burstow maintains that texts are not always explicitly present in an encounter: "[T]exts profoundly influence practice *even when they are not purposefully activated*. Concepts like *family psychosis*, for example, lodge in our heads, dictate what we see" (Burstow 2015, pp. 18–19). Indeed, this seems an apt description of what Ikma and Janet were put through by the CNO, as implicitly informed by the *Diagnostic and Statistical Manual of Mental Disorders* (DSM). No edition of it was ever named in either of the interviews, nor was any similar publication that describes what "depression" or "bi-polar disorder" is. Yet, surely the DSM ultimately dictates what was taken-for-granted in the processes to which Ikma and Janet were subjected. If nothing like the DSM existed, none of what Ikma and Janet experienced from the College would have been possible.

Every single activation and granting of agency discussed previously can be traced back to the DSM and its institutionalization of the idea of "mental illness," of some people as objectively knowable and distinguishable as "depressed" or "bi-polar," of such designations amounting to a kind of medicalized failure to be fully functioning humans, of psychiatry as the appropriate authority on such matters, and so forth. The DSM was activated, in both stories, the very moment the initial disclosure was made. After years of "competent" practice, having seemingly only ever been viewed as a competent practitioner, all it took was the uttering of "depression" or "bi-polar" in the wrong conversation and everything fell apart.

That said, if Burstow's example of "family psychosis" lends itself well to understanding the role played by "depression" and "bi-polar" in the stories, we are not sure that the same is true of the immediate and local operation of anti-Black racism in Ikma's story. There are many textual instances of anti-Black racism that reiterate the suggestion that young Black women are incompetent, irresponsible, dangerous, too emotional, and so on; but is there anything that plays a role parallel to that played by the DSM in relation to sanism? We could check the archives of the local papers and would likely find racist accounts of the festival whose traffic delayed Ikma, but those articles would be no more *a source* for her colleague's racism than any number of other texts or non-textual iterations of racism we could identify.

So, if the DSM was an "absent presence" once the complaint against her went from behavioral to constitutional (i.e., who she is rather than what she did), what does it mean that no analogous text can be identified as the ultimate authoritative source of anti-Black racism? Does it suggest that some things lend themselves to strict institutional ethnography more than others? Might IE contain an implicit bias toward power relations that are explicitly and traceably textually mediated? Might this even mean that it is not so well suited to forms of oppression, such as racism, sexism, and homophobia, that are less likely to leave a paper trail because they are (erroneously) widely hailed as a thing of the past and not bureaucratized? What about neoliberalism can account for why both nurses found themselves in such precarious employment settings, given the trend both nationally and globally toward precarity across sectors (Klein 2001)? Even a key text, such as the North American Free Trade Agreement, still does not serve a function in neoliberalism quite like that of the DSM in psychiatry. Might the insistence on texts steer researchers away from some kinds of structural violence?

Regardless, institutional ethnography provides compelling ways to concretely trace power relations. Besides if we look to an early study called "K Is Mentally Ill" that Smith (1978) did before naming and (dare we say) "institutionalizing" IE, we find how helpful IE-like practices are even in tracing non-textual workings of power.

In "K Is Mentally Ill," Smith noted that people may initially be defined as "mentally ill" through social relations outside of "the activities of the official agencies" that deal with "mental illness" (1978, p. 24). She traces the construction of K as "mentally ill" through a careful analysis of an interview that was done with one of K's friends about K, and she notes that other researchers too have found "that a good deal of non-formal work has been done by the individual concerned, her family, and friends, before entry to the official process" of psychiatrization (1978, p. 24).

Smith's "Anatomy" of a Person's Disqualification

In tracing the construction of K as "mentally ill," Smith writes:

> The alternative picture, very simply stated, was that what was going on was a kind of communal freezing-out [or ostracization] process ... and that if there was anything odd in K's behaviour (and reading the account suggested to me that there was doubt whether anything *was* very psychiatrically odd) it might reasonably be supposed that people do react in ways which seem odd to others when they are going through this kind of process [i.e., where their peers collectively and cumulatively ostracize them]. (1978, pp. 25–26)

Smith's analysis of how she had been initially convinced of K's mental illness is a brilliant example of the kind of work she would later describe as documenting "discourse as an actually happening, actually performed, local organizing of consciousness among people" (2001, p. 177). Also this study lends itself nicely to an exploration of what took place with both Janet and Ikma on the job before the official complaints to the College were made. Like K, to whatever extent Janet and Ikma could be said to have acted "odd," any of this can easily be explained by the distressing situations they found themselves in at the workplace—and therefore as a response to neoliberal job precarity, sanism, and/or racism.

In Janet's story, she returned to her 12-step program after many years of sobriety, and she requested to shorten her shifts. These are signs of self-care rather than pathology, but we can assume she was struggling. However, there are any number of explanations that can be called on to make sense of this struggle. Jerry understood it as a problem in terms of who Janet is—an "addict" and a "depressive." Janet, though, situated the initial increase in stress as being relocated from a workplace where she had been comfortable, engaged, and respected for decades to a new setting with a new supervisor and "desk job" responsibilities that she was not enthusiastic about. Her reassignment was because of an amalgamation, not because of anything Janet had done wrong, and we can assume that the hospital needed to place her somewhere and there happened to be room for a nurse in an office job.

Such transitions and loss of control over one's work life are commonly held to be sources of difficulty for people. In addition, there is no indication that Jerry or anyone else interpreted Janet's difficulties as anything other than "normal" transition concerns and displeasure with a new role she had not chosen—that is, until Janet spoke the word "depression" to Jerry.

Tellingly, in Ikma's story, she left her shift early, not having completed a procedure with a patient, just as the initial letter from the College stated. She said in her interview that she wishes the complaint had been left at that because likely she would have been placed on probation, at worst. Also if she had been given a real chance to tell her side of the story, she may not even have been reprimanded at all. Her colleagues and de facto supervisors were not acting according to standardized protocol (i.e., in relation to both safety and compliance with the law) in several ways, and they directed her to do the same. Remember too that she was in a precarious situation as a casual employee, so a reprimand for breaching protocol could have been anticipated to potentially cost Ikma her job. She was in a fairly impossible situation when she left her shift early.

Further, we can speculate that Ikma may have shown up for her shift feeling frazzled after being delayed and then getting lost. Again, this is an expected human response to such a situation, especially on one's first day of a new job. Then too, we can imagine further that if she then found that they believed she had been out partying the night before (as an explanation to why she was late), and that she, like most people, would also have found this distressing—all the more so again when this appeared to be motivated by assumptions grounded in anti-Black racism. It is no surprise that this was a difficult day for her. If anything, it would be odd if it had not been.

Both Janet and Ikma found themselves being treated analogously to how K was treated by her friends, which Smith described as an ostracization or "communal freezing-out process." In Ikma's story, racism seems to have been animating her colleague's mistreatment of her that day, initially fleshing out the story of her as late/lost to a story of her as intrinsically unreliable and undesirable; in Janet's story it was sanism from the point that she mentioned her past diagnosis to Jerry. In both situations, though, we can imagine that their distress would have understandably increased as a result of their colleagues' harassment: refusing to help and directing her to go against protocol in Ikma's case; scrutiny, distrust, and surveillance in Janet's.

Again, there may well have been an increase of behavior that their colleagues interpreted as "odd," but, as Smith reminds us, "it might reasonably be supposed that people do react in ways which seem odd to others when they are going through this kind of process." So Ikma left her shift early, feeling that she could not do what the other nurses were directing her to do and surely feeling very unsafe about how she was being treated. Janet, for her part, may also have become more upset in response to the surveillance, but again this would be expected given what Jerry was putting her through.

From the time of Jerry's harassment of Janet and the seemingly, at the point of after-the-fact interpretation, of Ikma (her initial letter from the College made no mention of it), all of their behavior was read through the lens of "mental illness." We are not touching on the question of whether the Ikma and Janet diagnoses are real (as applied to them, or as applied to anyone). They have their own understandings of that—Janet feeling she should be accommodated as she would if she had any other illness; Ikma questioning whether she really *is* "bipolar"—and as a research team, we likely represent somewhat diverse analyses of such things too. But, like Ikma and Janet, we are all certain that whatever "mental illnesses" they might or might not have had and whether the concept does or does not have any validity, it had nothing at all to do with the "freezing out" of the profession that they experienced. Whatever the "reality" of their "brain chemistry," they were both constructed as mentally ill within a discourse and structure that conflates "mental illness" with unreliability, danger, deficit, and incompetence in everyday and work life.

Smith writes that it "is not clear what norms are deviated from when someone is categorized as mentally ill" (1978, p. 26), and yet people seem to arrive at conclusions about others' "mental illness" with curious certainty. Jerry believed that Janet's depression was a cause of concern, so recruited Janet's colleagues to document supporting evidence using their subjective judgments and interpretations—perhaps knowing of Janet's diagnosis, perhaps not. Ikma was racially framed as unreliable when she finally arrived at work that day, likely already flustered. When she requested support from her colleagues, they either discriminatingly "froze her out" or did so perhaps assuming she was undesirable as a nurse. Either way, Janet's and Ikma's colleagues conflated interpretations of "incompetence" as truth.

We can also imagine that both nurses were being measured in relation to norms of which they might not have been aware. Regarding K, the example Smith uses is that of the swimming pool. K's friend Angela, who told the story to the interviewer, said that others "would sort of dip in and just lie in the sun, while K insisted that she had to swim 30 lengths ... [so that, according to Smith] Angela's beach behaviour provides the norm in terms of which K's behaviour is to be recognized as deviating" (1978, p. 34) rather than K being seen as "athletic."

In relation to Janet and Ikma, they were both working in unfamiliar hospital settings. Perhaps protocol was broken routinely in Ikma's hospital, making her refusal to do so appear "odd," but we can hardly assume it is a common norm and, more important, the risk to a contract nurse outweighs a unionized one. Working in the same hospital for decades, Janet knew the people and procedures with the kind of rigor that only comes from an extended period of immersion. When she was in a new environment she was not recognized as an expert trainer, researcher, scholar, and care provider. Janet too may have taken norms for granted from the previous administration, which were not standard in the new hospital environment.

As a result of these kinds of processes, where an interpretation becomes fact and a person's actions are constructed as "incompetent" when deviating from a norm, those who are granted institutional agency to speak the truth "produce for themselves and others what they can recognize as rational and objective. It is the *recognition* of what is said and done that produces it as accountably accomplishing the rationality and objectivity of a given institutional order" (Smith 2001, pp. 182–183). That is to say, these narrative devices enable a misrecognition of something as true.

Reflecting on her initial perception of K as mentally ill, Smith suggests that "something like a 'willing suspension of disbelief' effect is operating—that is, I tended to suspend or bracket my own judgemental process in favour of that of the teller of the tale" (1978, p. 34). We can assume that something like this would have been in effect for many of those granted agency to discredit and disqualify Ikma and Janet. When they were presented with one person's account of their new colleague as needing to be observed, or as irresponsible, they tended to favor that interpretation over their own so that Ikma and Janet then appeared to them to be just that. Such a framing is self-perpetuating in that it propagates what is clearly a biased and one-sided story. As a result, as Smith writes:

> [It] ought not to be a problem for the reader/hearer who properly follows the instructions for how the account is to be read [i.e., that this person *is* "mentally ill"], that no explanation, information, etc., from K is introduced at any point in the account. And it is not or ought not to be strange that at no point is there any mention of K being asked to explain, inform, etc. In sum then, the rules, norms, information, observations, etc., presented by the teller of the tale are to be treated by the reader/hearer as the only warranted set. ... The actual events are not facts. It is the use of proper procedure for categorizing events which transforms them into facts. (1978, p. 35)

It is the framing of Janet and Ikma as "mentally ill" (conflated with "incompetent") that enabled the CNO to disregard their alternate accounts of events, their legitimate grievances, and assertions of their "competence." What Smith calls "the use of proper procedure" transformed sanist accounts into facts. No alternative explanation was admissible into the "factual account" that had been created and perpetuated. Whether certain texts were activated or not, and certain persons were granted agency or not, this would all have taken place in accordance with a logic in which it had already been determined what would and would not count as fact.

Nonetheless, it is actually a little worse than simply not taking up alternate facts. Ikma's and Janet's actions and reactions are not only disregarded as non-facts; they may instead become taken up as evidence against them. In the example of K at the pool, it is not simply that her athleticism (mentioned several times in the account of her) is erased from the vignette; this very likely motivation for her actions is substituted for an explanation of her as a fixed kind of person—"mentally ill"—so that 30 lengths is not a testament to her as hardworking and athletic. Neither can it be an indication that perhaps she is stressed to be hanging out with friends who are increasingly ostracizing and othering her; it is, instead, a "symptom." No need of further interrogation required.

Smith connects this to a "medical model" framing of people in which "behaviour is treated as arising from a state of the individual and not as motivated by features of her situation" (Smith 1978, p. 38). Such fixed-state understandings of what it is to be human are typical of psychiatric and psychological framings, whereas outside of these discourses, people have tended to understand that fellow humans do what they do in response to their context and as guided by values, commitments, and intentions (Chapman 2012, p. 148).

The difference between framing someone as motivated by their values and in response to a particular context, on the one hand, and as motivated by a fixed inner (pathological) state, on the other, is enormous. It is perhaps even the crux of the difference between whether someone is competent to live, evaluate and discern, and practice a complex task such as nursing. Readers may have gotten to this point and still be thinking that Ikma clearly, after all, did leave her shift and the patients for which she was entrusted to care. This is true, but how we frame it makes all the difference in the world. The case has been made against her that she is "incompetent" because she is "bi-polar," as a complete explanation for her actions that day. That is one story that can be told, and it has had disastrous consequences.

But if Ikma's day was one in which she was facing racism and clearly reprimandable unethical practice from her colleagues, then perhaps walking out was a principled decision—a way of communicating that what they were doing (i.e., to her and more generally in their nursing practice) was not acceptable. Then if that is the case, surely she is precisely the kind of person we want caring for us and our loved ones in a hospital—a person who will do what is right, who will take a stand, even if the local organizational culture is racist and unethical.

At the very least, we have to ask ourselves what on earth is going on when taking a stand in such a way is so easily understood as psychopathology and, therefore, as a reason for someone to be prevented from ever nursing again? We need to ask what purpose it really serves to imagine "mental illness" as a reason that a person should not help others, and how it is that mental illness is so easily conflated with "incompetence"?

NOTE

1. This chapter is part of an ongoing research project and our collaboration on it only occurred because Bonnie brought us together with this book in mind. Thank you, Bonnie.

REFERENCES

Abdillahi, I., Meerai, S., & Poole, J. (in press). When the suffering is compounded: Towards anti-Black sanism. In S. Wehbi & H. Parada (Eds.), *Re-imagining anti-oppression: Reflections on practice*. Waterloo: Wilfrid Laurier Press.

Alaers, J. (2010). Two-spirited people and social work practice: Exploring the history of Aboriginal gender and sexual diversity. *Critical Social Work, 11*(1). Retrieved from: http://www1.uwindsor.ca/criticalsocialwork/two-spirited-people-and-social-work-practice-exploring-the-history-of-aboriginal-gender-and-sexual-d

Aronson, J., & Hemingway, D. (2011). "Competence" in neoliberal times: Defining the future of social work. *Canadian Social Work Review, 28*(2), 281–285.

Benjamin, A. (2003). *The Black/Jamaican criminal: The making of ideology*. Unpublished doctoral dissertation, University of Toronto, Toronto.

Birnbaum, M. (1960). The right to treatment. *American Bar Association Journal, 46*, 499–505.

Birnbaum, R., & Silver, R. (2011). Social work competencies in Canada: The time has come. *Canadian Social Work Review, 28*(2), 299–303.

Bogo, M., Mishna, F., & Regehr, C. (2011). Competency frameworks: Bridging education and practice. *Canadian Social Work Review, 28*(2), 275–279.

Burstow, B. (2015). *Psychiatry and the business of madness: An ethical and epistemological accounting*. New York: Palgrave Macmillan.

Callow, E. (2013). The Indian Child Welfare Act: Intersections with disability and the Americans with Disabilities Act. *Clearinghouse Review: Journal of Poverty Law and Policy, 46*, 501–539.

Campbell, C. (2011). Competency-based social work: A unitary understanding of our profession. *Canadian Social Work Review, 28*(2), 311–315.

Canadian Council of Social Work Regulators. (2013). http://www.ccswr-ccorts.ca/index_en.html

Carignan, L. (2011). Les référentiels de compétences sont-ils un outil pour les organismes régulateurs et une commande pour les milieux de formation? *Canadian Social Work Review, 28*(2), 287–293.

Chamberlin, J. (1990). The ex-patients' movement: Where we've been and where we're going. *Journal of Mind and Behavior, 11*(3/4), 323–336.

Chapman, C. (2012). Colonialism, disability, and possible lives: The residential treatment of children whose parents survived Indian residential schools. *Journal of Progressive Human Services, 23*(2), 127–158.

Chapman, C. (2013). Cultivating a troubled consciousness: Compulsory sound-mindedness and complicity in oppression. *Health, Culture and Society, 5*(1), 182–198.

Fook, J. (2011). The politics of competency debates. *Canadian Social Work Review, 28*(2), 295–298.

Klein, N. (2001). *No logo*. New York: Picador.

Mills, C. (2014). *Decolonizing mental health: The psychiatrization of the majority world*. New York: Routledge.

Perlin, M. L. (1992). On sanism. *Southern Methodist University Law Review, 46*, 373–407.

Poole, J., & Ward, J. (2013). Breaking open the bone: Storying, sanism and mad grief. In B. LeFrançois, R. Menzies, & G. Reaume (Eds.), *Mad matters* (pp. 94–104). Toronto: Canadian Scholars Press.

Poole, J., Jivraj, T., Arslanian, A., Bellows, K., et al. (2012). Sanism, "mental health" and social work/education: A review and call to action. *Intersectionalities: A Global Journal of Social Work Analysis, Research, Polity and Practice, 1*, 1, 20–36.

Reid, J., & Poole, J. (2013). Mad students in the social work slassroom? Notes from the beginnings of an inquiry. *Journal of Progressive Human Services, 24*(3), 209–222.

Rossiter, A., & Heron, B. (2011). Neoliberalism, competencies, and the devaluing of social work practice. *Canadian Social Work Review, 28*(2), 305–309.

Smith, D. E. (1978). "K is mentally ill": The anatomy of a factual account. *Sociology, 12*(1), 23–53.

Smith, D. E. (2001). Texts and the ontology of organizations and institutions. *Studies in Cultures, Organizations and Societies, 7*(2), 159–198.

Todd, S. (2011). Competencies: Introduction. *Canadian Social Work Review, 28*(2), 273–274.

Widerberg, K. (2004). Institutional ethnography—Towards a productive sociology. An interview with Dorothy E. Smith. *Sosiologisk Tidskrift, 12*, 179–184.

CHAPTER 4

Spirituality Psychiatrized: A Participatory Planning Process

Lauren J. Tenney in consultation with Celia Brown,
Kathryn Cascio, Angela Cerio, and Beth Grundfest-Frigeri

SETTING THE SCENE

The subject of this chapter is not research that I have done and completed but the process of coming to a research topic and the beginnings and early ideas of a research team that coalesced to explore the issue. The project takes as its problematic the psychiatrization of people as a result of their spiritual experiences. How is it, I asked, that people find themselves ripped from a life, which includes spiritual experiences, and transported, generally forcibly, into the psychiatric system?

Just before Dr. Bonnie Burstow[1] released her call for proposals for this anthology, I became engrossed in a cable television series entitled "The Ghost Inside My Child" (see http://www.imdb.com/title/tt3107588/). The general point of the series was attempting to establish validity and evidence for the reports of children at least seemingly having access to previous life stories

L.J. Tenney (✉)
Staten Island, NY, USA
e-mail: TenneyPhDMSU@gmail.com

C. Brown
Bronx, NY, USA

K. Cascio
Albany, NY, USA

A. Cerio
Staten Island, NY, USA

B. Grundfest-Frigeri
Far Rockaway, NY, USA

© The Editor(s) (if applicable) and The Author(s) 2016
B. Burstow (ed.), *Psychiatry Interrogated*,
DOI 10.1007/978-3-319-41174-3_4

or past lives. Several of the stories addressed were based on interviews with the child and parents or other adults in the child's life. What was portrayed with varying details, at some point over the course of what otherwise would have been ordinary daily events, were children describing to their parents or other adults remembered scenes from different places and times, none of which would be accessible to the child through her or his environment. Some of the children spotlighted on the show were toddlers. They were at a developmental stage of just acquiring language. Other young people featured on the show were teens. Spotlighted teenagers shared with viewers what struck them, as well as some around them, as types of past life memories, which they had initially had in early childhood.

These reported flashbulb memories that children had—with no explanation for the knowledge of other worlds at least seemingly imparted to them through the experiences—sometimes seemed comforting to those who experienced them, but often unsettled or terrified the children. The fear and terror appeared to stem from what they described as remnants of lives ended too quickly because of violence, illness, accident, or some other unforeseen tragic happening. A mix of historians and other professionals, and often the parents themselves, is shown throughout the episodes digging about on the Internet and in historical archives, such as digitized newspapers or maps; sometimes revisiting the actual places the children describe is included, thus trying to make meaning of what young children are saying about these worlds from afar. Viewers are shown the places and often the children themselves go back to the physical locations with their families for some type of closure of their past lives.

Perhaps you are dismissing the possibilities explored in this show as examples of madness. To me, this was at once a highly meaningful and credible series for what was presented intersects with my own beliefs. My interests and beliefs, I would add, sometimes cause discomfort for others when they learn of them. Then again, and perhaps more to the point, I know the insides of a psychiatric institution, in part because of my interests and beliefs, referred to by the doctor as "magical thinking." This magical thinking was used, in part, as justification for my "psychiatric assignment." As I watched the shows, I would wonder: What would have happened if instead of naming my situation as "psychiatric," someone had adopted a spiritual perspective? My point here is that my own experiences of being forcibly involved with psychiatry act as a motivating factor for taking on this work.

The second motivating factor came from the aforementioned television program episode, where a mother made mention of the debate she had with others with whom she discussed her child's behavior, in this case that included intense night terrors and resulted in the child refusing to go to sleep. The suggestion given to her by a coworker (a clinician) was to bring a psychiatrist in to evaluate the radical shift in the child's behavior—to assess the fear and anxiety. The mother on this show was concerned that if she took this psychiatric avenue, they would "diagnose" (label) and "medicate" (drug) her child.

At the time, an "Introduction to Psychology" course I was teaching included an assignment on conducting a literature search on something each student was interested in learning more about within the field of psychology. I also did the assignment along with the students and what I chose to search for was a combination of "past lives," "memory," and "reincarnation." The searches returned hundreds of articles about past life memories and reincarnation. Indeed, as I found, there is a rich academic literature on past lives and reincarnation. I remember feeling both surprise and satisfaction with this reality. Students also displayed a mixture of intellectual and emotional responses when I conducted these searches in front of them.

The literature based on past life memories and reincarnation, each from multiple perspectives, offers pro and con arguments for the existence of reincarnation. Although no article I came across establishes convincing evidence for past lives, some built a case for its plausibility. The cultural differences that surfaced are especially telling.

The point is, cultural hegemony would have to be suspected in the automatic rejection of past life experiences found in the West, for in many non-Judeo-Christian religions and cultures the concept of reincarnation is a fundamental part of the belief system. Masayuki Ohkado (2013), on the faculty of General Education at Chubu University in Aichi, Japan, and the Division of Perceptual Studies at the University of Virginia in Charlottesville, Virginia, delved specifically into one situation of what is termed "Cases of the Reincarnation Type (CORT)" (p. 625). Ohkado detailed the experiences of a young Japanese boy, Tomo, and referred to the earlier work of Dr. Ian Stevenson and others who:

> ...found more than 2700 cases of children who claim to remember their past lives from all over the world, including India, Thailand, Burma, Lebanon, Turkey, Sri Lanka, the UK, France, Germany, The Netherlands, Italy, Austria, Portugal, Hungary, Iceland, Finland, Canada, and the United States of America. (p. 625)

Ohkado (2013) was excited to contribute the story of Tomo, who by the time he was four was communicating about a previous life he had lived in Edinburgh, Scotland. Ohkado included a footnote explaining that Tomo was seen by a "psychiatrist, who diagnosed him with Asperger's Syndrome" (p. 635) because of his behavior and actions in relation to his past life memories. Thinking about Ohkado's work brought me back to my original concern presented by the mother in "The Ghost Inside My Child"—a mother fearing that a psychiatric response to her child's lived experience would leave her child at risk of being "diagnosed" and drugged. In fact, this is the exact position taken by most psychiatrists. They regularly admit that the field has no "cures" but does have "medications" that may alleviate the "symptoms" described or "observed."

What psychiatry fails to tell people, of course, is that the "symptoms" to which they refer are the result of being human in an often capitalist, survive-or-die environment that is both powered and protected by the State. I immediately became angry. Is there nowhere safe from psychiatry? Although not the same as my own situation, this struck me as akin to an injustice I experienced. When I described a spiritual experience to a psychiatric worker, note, it was reacted to as if it were a disease that required drugs.

The third factor that propelled me, and probably the most relevant one, was one finding of the (de)VOICED research project (GC CUNY IRB 400598-4, Tenney 2014). (de)VOICED showed that people's experience of spiritual, religious, or other altered states of consciousness are psychiatrized—the word *psychiatrized* being the shorthand for a subsequent course of involvement with psychiatry not only without informed consent but also over their expressed objection (for a discussion of this term, see LeFrançois and Coppock 2014).

By way of information, (de)VOICED: Human Rights Now (Tenney 2014) was an Environmental Community-Based Participatory Action Research Project that involved more than 100 people; an international planning effort; national data collection, where we used video to collect our data; and an extensive evaluation by 30 experts in the field of psychiatric systems change. The participants in the study created environmental "workographies" about their experiences working in an "outed" position of someone who has a psychiatric history.

(de)VOICED was evaluated in December 2012. People who participated in the evaluation also regarded the psychiatrization of spirituality as a problem—and it was something slated for future research. Subsequently, I received Bonnie Burstow's announcement about her institutional ethnography (IE) book project, which included a description of the subject and an offer of training. Correspondingly, after attending her workshops, I began viewing the IE method as a promising one for mapping out precisely how the psychiatrization of spirituality happens.

The final motivator was the recent US Legislative Hearings (2014) on the controversial "Murphy Bill," HR 3717, the "Helping Families in Mental Health Crisis Act." In these hearings, Congressman Murphy offered the "reality" of people believing they were "the angel Gabriel or Jesus" as proof for why his controversial, pro-forced-psychiatry law was necessary.

Four motivations then were involved in my responding to Burstow's call for proposals for this book, *Psychiatry Interrogated*. First, I wanted to explore my own experiences of psychiatric workers using my spiritual experiences against me and as grounds for psychiatric assignment. Second, I wanted to further my knowledge about research looking at children's reports of past lives either being taken as spiritual or psychiatrized. Third, and most relevant to conducting research, are the stories of the people who participated in (de)VOICED. It was inspiring to hear people courageously describe their spiritual and religious experiences as at the root of why they were assigned a psychiatric diagnosis and forcibly made to comply with a psychiatric regimen.

Correspondingly, the question that presented itself was: How can we show that the psychiatrization of spirituality is an institutional phenomenon and not a collection of isolated incidents? Finally, the fourth motivator for this work was the use of people believing themselves to be religious figures, or those around them to be devils, as justification in US legislative hearings for pro-force legislation.

Admittedly, much too ambitiously, based on the preceding happenings, I submitted a proposal for a joint piece of research on how it is that spirituality is psychiatrized. I reached out to others, mainly American psychiatric survivors with similar experiences, interested in pursuing this question.

It is important to underscore that this chapter is not purporting to reveal results of new research. Rather, it highlights a discussion based on a participatory planning process among people with a concern for the way in which psychiatry treats spiritual and religious experiences. Through this planning process, my collaborators and I have been working toward producing a plan for conducting research that will (hopefully) allow us to show how psychiatry turns people's spiritual beliefs into evidence of "mental illness" and justification for psychiatric intervention.

To be clear, we originally thought that together we would do the research in question in time to get into this book. As time passed, it became apparent that the project in question was beyond what we would be able to do in time, and that I would solo author a piece for the anthology about our processes and thoughts to date.

COLLABORATORS

To secure collaborators who would walk this journey with me, I put out an open call to my networks via Facebook and invited members of the (de) VOICED Research Team to participate in this process. As a way of facilitating this, I set up a private Facebook group (meaning only members of the group could find, see, or participate in it).

Hereafter, quotations in this chapter not otherwise identified should be seen as coming from members of this Facebook group. The group page was established to create a virtual place to hold an ongoing dialogue on the topics of developing a Research Design and an Institutional Review Board Application Response for a Future "Study" (interrogation) of the "business/institution of psychiatry" (Burstow 2015, p. 3), as it reigns over the concepts of spirituality and/or religion.

To my delight, more than a dozen people responded, wanting to actively participate (and more showed support by "liking" various posts on my public Facebook timeline). I added people who responded affirmatively to my invitation to the private Facebook group. The people who participated in this planning process (through this private group) mostly identify as people with psychiatric histories. Some consultants in this group are interested in the subject because of a personal spiritual or religious experience she or he had—that is, being taken as grounds for psychiatrization. Here began our conversation about creating a research design to show how the spiritual or religious experiences of some people result in psychiatric involvement.

I set up the Facebook group in October of 2014. Since its inception participation has been limited, but meaningful. Phone calls I have had via group teleconferencing and on an individual basis have been extraordinarily helpful in defining and then locating the scope of the work that is getting done through this planning process.

INSTITUTIONAL ETHNOGRAPHY: MY STANDPOINT AND ENTRY INTO THE RESEARCH

My standpoint, my entry into the research, is as someone who 28 years ago was involuntarily institutionalized and drugged in New York, at least in part because of my spiritual experiences. My ultimate disjuncture is precisely that psychiatrization. The question that I am asking is how does psychiatry operate so that such disjunctures or violations occur? That is, how does it turn people's spiritual leanings into a warrant for both initial and ongoing psychiatrization?

In searching for guidance, I found an article in which Widerberg (2004) interviewed Dorothy E. Smith, the originator of institutional ethnography. Smith is quoted by Widerberg as clarifying the concept of standpoint as follows:

> Women's standpoint, as I have interpreted it, means starting in the real world. The social can only happen here. You have to find some way to explore the social as it actually happens. Every aspect of society is something that happens. So when I was looking for a way to approach knowledge and to consider the forms of knowledge—not as something that is in people's heads—I was looking for knowledge as something taking place in the actual social organisation among people, in the social relations. (p. 2)

Applying my own identity, my woman's standpoint, I substituted the standpoint of people who have a psychiatric history and have an interest in how spirituality is psychiatrized. The original abstract entitled "Spirituality on Trial: How Lawyers, Legislators, and Psychiatric Workers Use Spiritual Experiences to Push and Profit from a Pro-Forced-Psychiatry Agenda" was submitted to Burstow's call for proposals.

When thinking about "what happened," one thing that we came up with is that spiritual experiences are considered suspect—indicators of some supposed psychiatric label—by psychiatry, by legislators, and by lawyers involved with potentially removing freedoms from a person by court-ordering psychiatric evaluation. The suspicion of those who have spiritual experiences is that experiences outside the hegemonic are routinely being treated as something warranting involuntary involvement with psychiatry via court order, or lesser forms of coercion.

Such spiritual experiences, in essence, prompt psychiatric assignment and culminate in involuntary involvement with psychiatric practices, procedures, and products. In other words, reporting spiritual experiences to a psychiatric worker can be the prompt for psychiatric "treatment," and this can include "treatment" without informed consent, and even "treatment" over expressed objection. So then, as an advisor to this project reminds us, "they bill you for it."

Of particular interest as a follow-up to the (de)VOICED research, which in part focuses on a systems theory model, was what IE had to offer. In the interview Dorothy E. Smith gave to Karin Widerberg (2004), Widerberg asked Smith how institutional ethnography differs from systems theory. Smith responds:

> The frames of system[s] theory is the system under investigation, its understanding is confined in its own frame. Institutional ethnography, on the other hand, does not aim to understand the institution as such. It only takes the social activities of the institution as a starting point and hooking on to activities and relations both horizontal and vertical it is never confined to the very institution under investigation. Hereby the connections between the local and extra-local are made, making the workings of society visible. (p. 5)

Institutional ethnography provided us with a whole new way to go. What we now envisioned was a piece of research where the proposed participants—that is, the people that we intend to interview—were not people whose spiritual experiences were psychiatrized. Rather they were the people who, in their institutional roles, participate in the psychiatrizing of a spiritual situation—in other words, psychiatrists, lawyers, and legislators. It is our hypothesis that when asked how this process happens, people will routinely refer to certain texts, or what in IE is referred to as "boss texts." We believe there will be a pattern in responses, which we then will be able to show as inherent, pervasive, institutional, and structural in nature. We believe we will be able to hook what happens at a local level to an external location, often embedded in a text such as the DSM. In this regard, in the summation of her interview with Smith, Widerberg (2004) significantly comments:

> "Institutional Ethnography" signals an approach where the use of institutional texts in the co-ordinating of people's activities is being investigated, with the aim to illuminate how these are "hooked up"—as Dorothy E. Smith express[es] it— hierarchically and horizontally beyond that particular institution. An approach that connects or maybe rather cuts across so-called micro- and macro-levels by making the everyday world as problematic. (p. 7)

INITIAL DISCUSSIONS BY PEOPLE IN THE FACEBOOK GROUP

It was thought incredibly important to distinguish between religion and spirituality—thus this distinction initially occupied a good part of our conversations. Witness, in this regard, the following exchange on the Facebook group:

Angela: We need to define what we mean by "spirituality" as opposed to religious practices. To me "Spirituality" is a world view in which the essence of being is the source of unique personally meaningful experiences.

Beth: For me it's an expression of specific religious practices that allow my spirituality to be expressed. Indeed they can often be an expression of uniqueness and of cultural unity/identity at the same time. One specific example being the fact that I wear a Tallis (prayer shawl); at the moment I have two of them—both have bright and colorful decorations on them that to most would define them as definitely made for a female to wear. I also wear Tefilin at times during prayer. I'd take a guess that at least 30% of the Jewish community worldwide would say that I'm wrong to wear a Tallis as a female and about 50–60% would make the same judgment over my wearing/using my paternal grandfather's Tefilin. Of those who wouldn't just deem it wrong many would simply say that neither men nor women need to or should wear them at all.

Likewise, we discussed the history of people being seen as "mad" on the basis of spiritual beliefs. As Angela Cerio called me to say, she had heard on television that in the nineteenth century people were put into insane asylums for religious reasons. "Religious excitement" (Kirkbride 1850/1851, p. 173) was written as a reason for admission under "supposed cause of insanity in 1806 patients" in a table of raw data that was constructed by Dr. Thomas Kirkbride[2] on behalf of the Pennsylvania Hospital for the Insane. His Table VIII reflected the "supposed causes of insanity" (p. 173), included data (e.g., 38 "M" and 29 "F" and 67 "T"), and noted patients being institutionalized for "religious excitement" (p. 173[3]). "T" appears to mean "Total." In New York State, there were nine people institutionalized for "moral insanity" (p. 191). After probing such history, we began discussing assignment as key to the process.

PSYCHIATRIC ASSIGNMENT

Psychiatric assignment is the literal process of being evaluated and psychiatrically labeled, assigned a psychiatric diagnosis based on the DSM, choose your edition or perhaps you prefer one of Kraepelin's early editions. For an in-depth discussion of the invalidity of this process, see Burstow (2015).

Mapping State Texts

As we continued to discuss our study, we could quickly see that we were about to be involved, among other things, in mapping US state texts—in particular, the texts that govern the declaring of people as mad and the assigning of a diagnosis. In this regard, the boss text, the DSM and how it gets activated, was critical to our discussion (for details on the use of the DSM and its activation, see Burstow 2015). Nevertheless, we also discussed texts that attempt to engender cultural competence—and yet that themselves get caught up in, and so reinforce, the current knowledge regime.

Religiosity, spirituality, and understanding of spiritual beliefs ought to be core components of cultural competence. For decades, people with psychiatric histories have been insisting that such training be available. For better or worse (and indeed, as we have found, it has been both for better *and* for worse), the government has taken up some attempts. As an example, to contextualize our discussion, and to address Angela's request for a clear distinction between "religion" and "spirituality," I would like to look at the definitions supplied by this state-sponsored effort; and the process of government texts aiming to have the role of "boss texts" as per Dorothy Smith's IE method.

One such example is the *Clinician Guide to Enhancing Therapeutic Alliances for Members of Cultural Groups: Incorporating Religion and Spirituality* with its lead author Marta Herschkopf, MD, MSt (n.d.). This work was published by the Center of Excellence in Culturally Competent Mental Health at one of the New York State Office of Mental Health's research facilities, the Nathan Kline Institute. Broadening the understanding of psychiatric workers' ability to incorporate religion and spirituality is something people want. This is how culture, religion, and spirituality are defined in the *Clinician Guide* (n.d.):

Culture: The way of life for a group of people, encompassing behaviors, beliefs, values, and symbols passed along from one generation to the next.

Religion: An organized system of beliefs, practices, rituals, and symbols related to a search for the sacred or transcendent.

Spirituality: The belief that there is something greater than the physical world that provides a connectedness to the universe and to all its inhabitants.[4]

In another effort, The Center for Spirituality and Healthcare at the NYU Langone Medical Center and the NKI Center of Excellence in Culturally Competent Mental Health (Galanter et al. 2012) put forward a 51-page product aimed at psychiatric practitioners in a variety of clinical settings, referred to here as "A Group Leader Guide." The authors stated: "There is a growing openness to accepting the role of spirituality as an important component for patients coping with illness" (p. 6). They go on for dozens of pages explaining how to conduct spirituality groups, address problematics such as disruptive participants (p. 24), people who are dogmatic (p. 25), people who monopolize or do not talk at all (p. 26), and people who according to the authors inappropriately share trauma histories (p. 27). Galanter et al. discuss a variety of settings and types of groups in which to discuss spirituality, including psychiatric settings (pp. 33–35).

Under the heading "Psychiatric Setting," the authors are clear: "Spirituality is important to many psychiatric patients" (p. 33). They offer a "case vignette" (pp. 33–34) in which a man assigned the diagnosis "schizoaffective disorder" wants his rabbi and psychiatrist to meet (p. 33). In the vignette, the person confides in his rabbi about his psychiatric assignment and that he was involved with a psychiatrist. In the "A Group Leader Guide," it is explicitly stated:

The rabbi offered to speak with the psychiatrist and see if there were ways they could work together that would help [the person] feel that he could integrate his spirituality into his recovery. The member was excited at this thought but was also unsure as to how the psychiatrist would react. He did not want the psychiatrist to think he was crazy because he thought spirituality could help him with his illness. The rabbi assured him that he would do nothing to hurt him in the eyes of the psychiatrist. (pp. 33–34)

The psychiatrist welcomed the involvement of the rabbi, albeit he had never considered spirituality as a source of support, or hope, or healing, and then asked other members of the group whether they had spiritual experiences. It is also mentioned, however, that cultural values and beliefs *can prevent* certain groups from accepting a psychiatric assignment, because of:

...[the] stigma attached to mental illness and psychopharmacological treatment. Latino patients may be more reluctant to follow through on treatment regimens or even to accept a diagnosis or framing of an illness when based on the Western biomedical model. (p. 34)

The "A Group Leader Guide" specifies that "spirituality" can be a "helpful bridge between acceptance of treatment and framing the disease" (p. 34). Although this may seem like openness, we saw it as a questionable use of spirituality. The point here is that precisely by including spirituality this way, the Guide contributes to the psychiatrization of people.

Now from a psychiatric survivor standpoint, it is the fear of being forced onto a psychiatric drug regimen that often keeps people from speaking the truth about their experiences. One reason people fear being psychiatrized is because there are many life-threatening and life-altering problems associated with psychiatric drugs including, and specific to this research proposal, "reduced psychic/spiritual openness" (Hall 2012, p. 22). Currently, psychiatry claims that the drugs address a chemical imbalance. Nevertheless, Hall's *The Harm Reduction Guide for Coming Off Psychiatric Drugs* is clear that psychiatry can make no such claims:

Philosophers and scientists have debated for centuries over the "hard problem" of how consciousness arises from the brain and body. Is what gets called "mental illness" a social and spiritual question more than a medical one? Is being called "disordered' a political and cultural judgment? Psychiatry can make no credible claim to have solved the mystery of the mind–body relationship between madness. (p. 16)

The "A Group Leader Guide" (Galanter et al. 2012), nonetheless, provides clear guidelines for distinguishing between "acceptable" and "unacceptable" types of spirituality and religion and the acceptable and unacceptable mixing between psychiatry and religious leaders. In turn, immediately following, three special topics are addressed: (1) "psychotic patients" (pp. 34–35); (2) "disorganized participants" (p. 35), who needed boundaries to "settle down and remain in the group" (p. 35); and (3) suicidal participants, who should be "closely monitored" but may have a "unique experience to discuss the value of life" (p. 35). The authors suggest that "spiritual comfort" can be of assistance in suicidal types of situations, but clarify: "The group leader should discuss any concerns he or she has about a participant who appears to be suicidal with that person's primary mental health care professional" (p. 35).

The fact that within the Guide, a line is drawn between acceptable and unacceptable potential participants for spirituality groups, the fact that it differentiates between acceptable and unacceptable types of spiritual discussion, we feel, further solidifies the need for our research project. For example, the "A Group Leader Guide" specifically rejects the usefulness of spirituality groups for "psychotic patients":

> Severely psychotic participants may be problematic. Religious preoccupation or delusions incorporating religious figures can make it very difficult, if not impossible, to carry on a productive group. In such a case, it may be preferable for such a patient not to attend the group. (p. 34)

Although we were originally hopeful about the Guide and indeed, it does make important points about culture, the fact that "severely psychotic participants" (p. 34) are identified in this way is problematic. From a psychiatric survivor standpoint, all the "A Group Leader Guide" shows is how far "cultural competence" must still travel and the unfortunate way that biological psychiatry is still in charge.

In other ways, the authors of the private–public collaborative Guide illustrate exactly what it is this proposed research design is trying to understand; and how spiritual or religious experiences are psychiatrized, even stating that in the case of people with spiritual delusions, "it may be preferable for such a patient not to attend the group" (p. 34). Of course, this in itself is evidence of a sort that psychiatry still psychiatrizes spiritual experiences.

Problematizing "psychotic" (p. 34), "disorganized" (p. 35), and "suicidal" (p. 35) experience and postioning the experiences in question as unacceptable types of spiritual experience, the "A Group Leader Guide" misses an opportunity to unhook psychiatry and social meaning. Now when focusing explicitly on the ways in which people who are Latina/o experience spirituality and religion, the Guide clearly distances "culturally sanctioned experiences" from a "medical or psychiatric context":

> These background statistics and descriptions demonstrate that certain imagery such as divine healing and the power of the Holy Spirit are commonly accepted cultural beliefs. What may be interpreted as delusional in a medical or psychiatric context may be understood and appreciated as a culturally sanctioned experience within the context of Latino Catholicism. (p. 41)

Yet the same authors (Galanter et al. 2012) wrote, those with "religious preoccupation or delusions incorporating religious figures" should not attend spirituality groups (p. 34). Once someone has been psychiatrized, the general rules of practice are suspended even though the Guide states that if someone has a particular belief, those beliefs should not necessarily be "interpreted as delusional in a medical or psychiatric context" and "may be understood and appreciated as a culturally sanctioned experience" (p. 41).

The "A Group Leader Guide" (Galanter et al. 2012) or indeed anything making its own claim to be a boss text, we could see, did not illustrate cultural competence. Instead, what I sensed is that the state-sponsored efforts create and perpetuate these exact types of discrimination their original aim is to dislodge.

Making the Process Visible

With input from the Facebook group, I worked at making visible the process that we were unearthing. Figure 4.1 illustrates psychiatrization based on spiritual experience.

First, a person has a spiritual experience that makes others uncomfortable and prompts involvement with psychiatry. Second, based on such boss texts of psychiatry as the DSM, which include spiritual experiences in the symptoms of their shell terms of "schizophrenia" and "psychosis," a person is then psychiatrically assigned. This assignment sometimes prompts a person to be forcibly subjected to psychiatric practices, procedures, and products. Enter the American Psychiatric Association (APA). The APA itself acknowledged spiritual and religious issues as potentially caught up in overuse of diagnoses and so created a possibly more problematic category of "illness" called "spiritual and religious issues." This led to a task force for the DSM-V that subsequently strengthened a differential diagnosis and a billing code for spiritual and religious issues (Koenig 2011).

After decades of demand for state-sponsored psychiatry to create culturally competent programming, New York State takes on the task and misses the mark, actually directing practitioners to disallow some who have spiritual experiences from participating in the spirituality groups being established in psychiatric institutions. This culminates with a person having a spiritual experience being further ostracized, psychiatrized, as someone incapable of participating in a spiritual group because of their spiritual experience.

Turning to Guidance from User and Survivor Research

Books and articles that we examined and discussed include Campbell (1997) and "Taken Seriously: The Somerset Spirituality Project" (as discussed in Faulkner 2004). In her article, Jean Campbell (1997) details how people who identified as consumers/survivors were involved with the evaluation of the quality of "psychiatric care" (p. 357) in public mental health facilities. Included in this article was a review of early theoretic works on recovery, with recovery defined as "some form of spirituality or philosophy that gives hope and meaning to life" (p. 360).

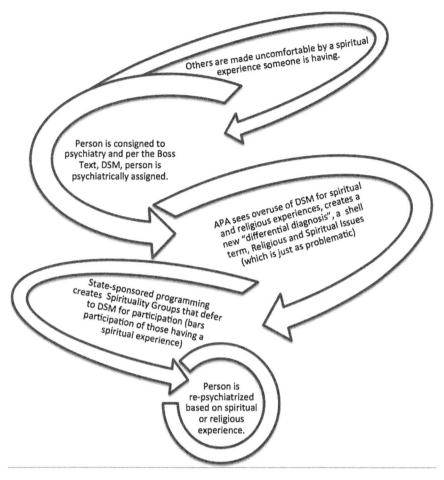

Others are made uncomfortable by a spiritual experience someone is having.

Person is consigned to psychiatry and per the Boss Text, DSM, person is psychiatrically assigned.

APA sees overuse of DSM for spiritual and religious experiences, creates a new "differential diagnosis", a shell term, Religious and Spiritual Issues (which is just as problematic)

State-sponsored programming creates Spirituality Groups that defer to DSM for participation (bars participation of those having a spiritual experience)

Person is re-psychiatrized based on spiritual or religious experience.

Figure 4.1   A map of how spiritual or religious experiences get psychiatrized.

The Taken Seriously Project is held up as an exemplar of survivor research in *The Ethics of Survivor Research: Guidelines for the Ethical Conduct of Research Carried Out by Mental Health Service Users and Survivors* (Faulkner 2004, pp. 29–30). Because this current proposal is an application to conduct a type of survivor research, it is important to note that according to Faulkner, "[s]urvivor research should attempt to counter the stigma and discrimination experienced by survivors in society" (p. 7), so this goal is implicit in our design.

Details of Discussions and Planning Relevant to the Literature

As I moved through the academic literature base, the people advising me continued to send proposals for future research that I think deserve attention. For example, Beth suggested two potential designs:

Possible Scenario/Question: If spiritual needs for religious observance require that the person be allowed to abstain from eating and drinking during daytime hours but allow and create the need for the person to be able to do so during night time (8 pm to 6 am) hours would this modification be allowed? (Ramadan and Yom Kippur are the holidays that come to mind first but I know there are others.) *Proposal/Topic:* What if, for spiritual and/or religious purposes a patient was required to cover up [his or her] physical form more than the general population and/or wear specific garments either all day or during rituals, would [he or she] be allowed to do so? Or which ones would you (the staffer/doctor/nurse/psychiatrist) be comfortable allowing? Floor length skirts/dresses, Turban (Sikh) keffiyeh/Hijab (Muslim/Arab), hooded robe [and] sandals (Wiccan), Talit, Tefilin, Yarmulke/headcovering (Jewish)—I know I'm missing a few but...

What follows is an example of the intense, honest dialogue about these intersecting and separate entities of religion and spirituality that was held among the group:

Kathryn: I wonder if a person who is Muslim would be allowed to pray even if it made other "patients, staff" uncomfortable. What happens when someone states that God talks to them, or they hear the voice of God, Jesus, Buddha, etc...?

Angela: My line was "If Jesus was alive today, he would be found on a psychiatric ward?"

Beth: I was asked repeatedly why don't I use the exception of being "sick" to eat on Yom Kippur (I was ... an inmate at a psych prison/"hospital" during that year's Holy Day) kept it mild and said I needed the time to read the prayers and meditations for the holiday! They still demanded that I break the fast about 3 or 4 hours early or face another 12 hours without food and an added drug/prn – I was so drugged I couldn't do much of anything.... It's things like that and quite a few others that make me so passionate about this issue. I met ... one Witch/Wiccan person there who's only real problem seemed to be a different variety of abuses at home, I grew rather close to this person because we were the only people who were not Christian and truly trying to practice our faiths. It was the first time that I had met someone of that faith.

Ideas for the proposal of a design were quickly growing. The question was: If we were trying to find out how spirituality was psychiatrized, who ought to be recruited as participants? We created a poll with the following basic categories: People who had been psychiatrized for spiritual experiences, people who psychiatrized others for spiritual experiences, people who create the laws that allow for the psychiatrization of spiritual experience, students in any of these fields, none of these, or other. Now on the Facebook page itself the category "People who had been psychiatrized for spiritual experiences" had three "likes." Through conversations, however, we came to the conclusion that the people whom we ought to recruit were the ones actually doing it, not having it done to them. Therefore, we settled on recruiting people who are psychiatric workers, lawyers, legislators, and students in any of these fields.

Even though I was intent on trying to nail down a research design, values remained the core of what was discussed on the Facebook page. In response to a post I put up suggesting a series of scenarios discussed by Nixon, Hagen, and Peters (2010), which included references to God, the following dialogue occurred:

> **Angela**: Why do we need to call it "God"? I think that when I have spiritual experiences I'm communicating with entities who are as much a part of that which most people call God as we all are – but are no longer completely focused in our reality, or plane of existence. They can sometimes be very intrusive.
> **Lauren**: I don't think we have to call it "God" but from above, those were direct quotes from the article.... I am mixing up the design so that it has things that have been evidenced as having been labeled as psychosis, which people later re-claimed as spiritual AND the ideas that people have offered here as possible scenarios.
> **Celia**: I think we need to use God because there are some of us, believe in God. So we can't rewrite reality of some of our people.
> **Angela**: I'm not talking about leaving "God" out of the picture, Celia. It's just that what I thought of as God before my first "episode" was completely blown away by the magnitude of the experience. And I cannot imagine any MH [mental health] professional even suggesting that what I was experiencing had anything to do with God. A "spiritual experience" maybe. It occurs to me that maybe MH professionals should be trained in spiritual competency.

We decided it was important to actually talk with each other as opposed to randomly posting notes on the Facebook group. We agreed to participate collectively in a teleconference. As occurs whenever a researcher opens up the planning process to the ideas of others, the original intent and vision that one had often get lost in the realities of the responses from people who are giving advice about what each considered important.

To give you an idea of the breadth of interests advisors to this project had, here is the list of potential research projects that we were going to try to take on:

- Punished, Restrained, and In Trouble: Religious Practice and Spiritual Expression as Problematics
- The Right to Practice: What Is the Letter of the Law? Policy?
- Follow the Food: How Are Religious Eating Practices Psychiatrized, Nickeled and Dimed?
- Cross-Systems, Cross-Cultures: West Meets East
- Stifled Spiritual Awakenings: Psychiatrized, Drugged
- We Are Who We Are, Not Who the System Wants Us to Be: Cultural Competence—Law, Policy, Religion, and Spiritual Experiences
- Access to Traditional and Nontraditional Religious and Spiritual Leaders while Institutionalized
- What Is a Spiritual or Religious Experience?

How ever is one to come up with a design that meets such wild criteria?

After this incredibly powerful teleconference with those who agreed to advise me, I had to take a step back because, when I put out the call for involvement as an advisor, I imagined people would respond who had experiences and interests like my own. What I found, though, was why it was so important to split potential research designs per religion, or per spirituality. I posted the following for the Facebook group:

> *First Reflection:* The problem is as basic as it can get. The conversation is light years away from the scenarios I imagined. It almost confirms for me entirely [that] I ought not divulge what I thought would be at the heart of the issue: Messianic (Farber 2013), visionary experiences (Farber 1993), psychiatrized and drugged. Rather, some of the issues spotlighted are so commonplace, so pedestrian, so much more of a problematic than the basic experiences of religious practice, such as dietary restrictions are problematized; refusal of access to a religious leader of one's choosing; cultural competency; a law or policy? I am working on the research design.

Proposed Study

I cannot discuss with total clarity the study that we are in the process of devising, as we anticipate it including the use of deception. We also will be seeking anonymity for ourselves as researchers. That said, our proposed subject inclusion criteria is grounded in the framework of the study. As the study's intent is to look for institutional patterns of behavior that can be mapped out based on multiple scenarios presented to participants, we have decided to speak with a wide swath of professionals involved with the procedures leading to forced psychiatry.

Participants in this proposed study, we have determined, will be people with diverse backgrounds from within the following fields: psychiatry, psychology, mental health counseling, law, public service and/or elected officials, medical, and public psychiatric/mental/behavioral health policy and/or administration. Examples of potential recruitees include: licensed professionals or unlicensed professionals (e.g., with LSW or MSW, licensed psychologist or research psychologist), a trial lawyer or a lawyer who teaches at a law school, practicing or nonpracticing professionals (e.g., working, retired, or unemployed, in or out of the job market), advanced students (e.g., graduate and terminal degrees). We also thought it important to have participant exclusion criteria. People who are current or former students of any of the researchers or study coordinators, for example, will be excluded from taking part in the study.

There are to be several, potentially four rounds of participation. Each round would have decreasing levels of privacy and confidentiality, until the final round of participation that occurs entirely in public view, live-streamed, and video-recorded. Each round will use an assortment of methods to collect data, including: pencil and paper tests, which we have received permission to use; qualitative open-ended interviews; focus groups; and, finally, public presentations. Each round has the goal of unearthing each participant's position on their own religious and spiritual experiences and their views of the experiences of those whom have a psychiatric history, with whom they interact. We intend to ask each participant what they themselves would do if they were a "treating physician" or an "appointed counsel," and so on—for example, what they would activate, what texts they would create, who they would pass a particular document onto next.

Our future looks like this: Sometime soon, we will get to the point of submitting a research design for ethical review. Once accepted, we will go about collecting data that can be used to map out the ways in which spiritual and religious experiences are responded to by psychiatry. In our initial analyses, we will be looking for psychiatric responses that include misinformation, coercion, or court order. Within that data, we will look for lines where one can say exactly how and at which points spirituality is psychiatrized. The hope is that not only will we be able to map how the psychiatrization takes place, but that we also will be able to produce ideas for people to use preventively such as "Things to never say to a psychiatric worker" or "Things psychiatric workers consistently hear that will prompt forcible 'treatment' by them."

CONCLUDING REMARKS

In this chapter, I started with a disjuncture—which led me into a discussion of psychiatrization of spirituality. I announced the beginnings of a research project into the phenomenon, guided by institutional ethnography principles; and I proceeded to discuss how a team was gathered to conduct this research. The chapter culminated with details on Facebook discussions, early planning, and the beginnings of an application to an Institutional Review Board (IRB) for ethical review in order to conduct research with human participants. The question posed is: How is it that nonhegemonic spiritual beliefs get translated into a warrant for such profound interference?

This chapter and the research that it heralds begins to shed light on the "how."

NOTES

1. Dr. Bonnie Burstow's incredible academic and activist work is certainly complemented by her generous and gracious dedication to helping psychiatric survivors (including myself) be heard. I am extremely grateful for both her acceptance of this chapter's project and all the work she put into helping it take shape.
2. Much can be said about Kirkbride, and in other works I discussed that he laid out the guidelines for the construction of hospitals for the insane, a committee that he chaired, and why the layout of many institutions that are characteristic of mid-nineteenth-century American psychiatry are attributed to his work.
3. Kirkbride, T. S. (see References; digitized by Google at http://babel.hathitrust. org/cgi/pt?id=ucl.32106015837112;view=1up;seq=183.
4. See http://1ngyaa163ye68k149pkecjnx.wpengine.netdna-cdn.com/wp-content/ uploads/2016/01/Clinican-Guide-ETAMCG-140602.pdf.

REFERENCES

Burstow, B. (2015). *Psychiatry and the business of madness: An ethical and epistemological accounting.* New York: Palgrave Macmillan.
Campbell, J. (1997). How consumers/survivors are evaluating the quality of psychiatric care. *Evaluation Review, 21*(3), 356–363.
Farber, S. (1993). *Madness, heresy, and the rumor of angels: The revolt against the mental health system.* Chicago: Open Court.
Farber, S. (2013). *The spiritual gift of madness: The failure of psychiatry and the rise of the mad pride movement.* Rochester: Inner Traditions.
Faulkner, A. (2004). *The ethics of survivor research: Guidelines for the ethical conduct of research carried out by mental health service users and survivors.* Bristol: The Policy Press.
Galanter, M., Talbot, M. S., Demitis, H., McMahon, C., Dugan, T., & Oktay, D. (2012). Conducting multicultural spirituality discussion groups in behavioral health treatment settings: A Group Leader Guide. Center for Spirituality and Healthcare, NYU Langone Medical Center, Nathan Kline Institute for Psychiatric Research, and NKI Center for Excellence in Culturally Competent Mental Health. Retrieved on September 1, 2014, from http://1ngyaa163ye68k149pkecjnx.wpengine.netdna-cdn.com/wp-content/uploads/2016/01/spiritgrpmanual.pdf.
Hall, W. (2012). *The harm reduction guide to coming off of psychiatric drugs* (2nd ed.). New York: The Icarus Project and Freedom Center.
Herschkopf, M., & NKI Center of Excellence in Culturally Competent Mental Health. (n.d.). Clinician guide to enhancing therapeutic alliances for members of cultural groups: Incorporating religion and spiritualty. Orangeburg: Nathan Kline Institute (NKI) Center of Excellence in Culturally Competent Mental Health. Retrieved on July 29, 2015, from http://1ngyaa163ye68k149pkecjnx.wpengine.netdna-cdn.com/wp-content/uploads/2016/01/Clinican-Guide-ETAMCG-140602.pdf.
Kirkbride, T. S. (1851–1852). Article VII, Section 7. Report of the Pennsylvania Hospital for the Insane, for the year 1850. Physician to the Institution. Published by order of the Board of Managers (pp. 172–175). In *(1851–1852). Reports of hospitals for the insane. Journal of Insanity, 8,* 155–195. Reprinted 1965. Digitized by Google.
Koenig, H. G. (2011). Schizophrenia and other psychotic disorders. In J. Peteet, F. G. Lu, & W. E. Narrow (Eds.), *Religious and spiritual issues in psychiatric diagnosis: A research agenda for DSM-V* (pp. 31–52). Arlington: American Psychiatric Association Press.
LeFrançois, B., & Coppock, V. (2014). Psychiatrized children and their rights: Starting the conversation. *Children & Society, 28*(3), 165–171.
Nixon, G., Hagen, B., & Peters, T. (2010). Psychosis and transformation: A phenomenological inquiry. *International Journal of Mental Health Addiction, 8*(4), 620–635.
Ohkado, M. (2013). A case of a Japanese child with past-life memories. *Journal of Scientific Exploration, 24*(4), 625–636.
Somerset Spirituality Project Research Team, & Nicholls, V. (Ed.). (2002). Taken seriously: The Somerset spirituality project. London: The Mental Health Foundation. Retrieved January 29, 2015, from http://www.mentalhealth.org.uk/content/assets/PDF/publications/taken-seriously.pdf
Tenney, L. (2014). (de)VOICED: Human rights now. *Volumes I, II, and III.* Graduate Center, CUNY: Proquest.
Widerberg, K. (2004). Institutional ethnography: Towards a productive sociology—An interview with Dorothy E. Smith. *Sosiologisk Tidskrift, 12,* r 2. Retrieved on February 3,2015,from http://www.scribd.com/doc/193292666/Karin-Widerberg-Intervju-Med-Dorothy-Smith#scribd

Operation ASD: Philanthrocapitalism, Spectrumization, and the Role of the Parent

Mary Jean Hande, Sharry Taylor, and Eric Zorn

More than ever, people are talking about autism. It has become the "epidemic" that North Americans have come to understand as one of the leading afflictions of youth today, "affecting more children worldwide than Diabetes, Cancer, and AIDS combined" (Spectrum of Hope Foundation, Autism 2015, n.p.). In the United States it has become a national priority and a lucrative financial opportunity. In 2006, the US Senate and House of Representatives passed the "Combating Autism Act," which has since justified the spending of more than a billion dollars, not on supporting individuals diagnosed with autism or their families, but on eliminating autism altogether (McGuire 2015, 2016).

Later in 2008, the United Nations General Assembly inaugurated its first World Autism Awareness Day on Wall Street, with a number of resolutions aimed at aggressively addressing the problem of autism in the modern world (McGuire 2016). This money feeds a thriving industry of "autism spectrum disorder" (ASD) research and advocacy focused on "eliminating a disease." The self-proclaimed autistic community has protested these initiatives by targeting leading advocacy organizations such as the DSM-5 Diagnostic Criteria (2015), "Autism Speaks." They insist that such organizations marginalize and silence people diagnosed with autism and "do damage … to the lives of autistic people and those with other disabilities" (Autistic Self Advocacy Network 2014b).

Autism, Anne McGuire (2015) argues, is framed through these stories and cultural phenomena as something wholly abnormal, an aberrant form of humanity, or even fundamentally antagonistic to being a healthy human being. The American Psychiatric Association's fifth edition (2013) of the *Diagnostic*

M.J. Hande (✉) • S. Taylor • E. Zorn
Ontario Institute for Studies in Education, University of Toronto, Toronto, ON, Canada
e-mail: maryjeanelizabeth@gmail.com

© The Editor(s) (if applicable) and The Author(s) 2016
B. Burstow (ed.), *Psychiatry Interrogated*,
DOI 10.1007/978-3-319-41174-3_5

and Statistical Manual of Mental Disorders (DSM-5) has also shaped the story of autism by reconceptualizing it as a spectrum, thereby broadening the way it is diagnosed and understood. This new ASD diagnosis also opens up new opportunities for "treatment," caregiving, advocacy, *and* financial investment.

Although clearly not at the forefront of these changes, some parents have played an important role in pushing for changes—a process we call "spectrumization." In our research, we have found parents leading advocacy campaigns (see McGuire 2016) and sitting on strategic boards (e.g., spectrumofhope. ca/foundation/, autismspeaks.org/about-us/board-directors). Such parents are playing an increasingly important role in marketing new treatments (see sst-institute.net/ca/parents/) and creating for-profit treatment, research, and educational initiatives. This frames and structures ASD not only as an abnormality or threat to be eliminated but also a spectrum of opportunities for financial investment.

At the beginning of this investigation, all three authors were struck by the contradictory roles that some parents play in seeking out and even helping to develop privatized "therapeutic resources" for ASD, sometimes in ways that contradict the interests of those who have been diagnosed—and the wishes expressed by members of the autistic movement (Gruson-Wood 2014; McGuire 2016). The processes of spectrumizing ASD and the development of associated resources comes to dominate or rule the social experiences of the child in ways very commonly alienating and dehumanizing. Worst of all, these processes appear unavoidable, as though there are no alternatives to the ruling relations of ASD.

Yet, we also discovered that "parents" are far from a homogenous category; rather there are contradicting race and class interests among parents who shape the way ASD is activated. Wealthy, white, North American mothers and fathers are more commonly involved in active positions—sitting on boards, fundraising, and advocating for research and treatment. Meanwhile, working-class immigrants tend to be isolated from these roles and have significantly more difficulty with advocacy efforts (Getfield 2015). Instead, they activate the ASD diagnosis mostly as a means of accessing much-needed resources. Ultimately, all parents become "captured" by the ASD frame, actively reproducing these ruling relations, even as they fetter parents. Herein lies our entry point.

This chapter discusses this problematic by tracing parents' navigation of bureaucracies as they seek to care for or "treat" their children. We also trace these activities into the ruling relations of psychiatric "spectrumization" and the "financialization" of advocacy organizations and public institutions. With this in mind, we argue two things: (1) that ASD is socially, culturally, *and economically* formed through capitalist social relationships that are mediated through the everyday activities of parents of those diagnosed with autism every time they activate the ever-changing and highly political DSM; and (2) that a closer look at ASD advocacy, fundraising, support services, research, and therapeutic interventions can reveal a different story about ASD than that of pathology, tragedy, or threat. Rather, we reveal a material reality of capital venture or financial opportunity that brings together public schools, advocacy organizations, and private financial investments.

EPISTEMOLOGY

For this investigation, we conducted one interview with a working-class immigrant mother, whom we will call "Sofia"[1]; she has twin sons, "David" and "Anthony," both diagnosed with Asperger's Syndrome. This was not used as a case study per se but rather, in keeping with the epistemology of institutional ethnography (IE), the interview was an entry point into our investigation. Two of the authors' work experiences—Sharry Taylor's experience as a teacher working with children diagnosed with ASD in a public school system, and Mary Jean Hande's experience working as a disability activist and professional care provider for youth diagnosed as autistic—are among the more formidable entry points that inform our analysis. According to Dorothy Smith (2005), IE begins with "some issues, concerns, or problems that are real for people" (p. 32).

Our task as researchers is to clarify these issues, concerns, or problems and to use them as entry points that guide our line of inquiry. In the process we reveal social relationships and how they relate to an institutional order. Using this line of inquiry through our experiences and our interviews, we can show how, through human activity, ASD becomes diagnosed and "treated" in the contradictory ways described previously. We take as our problematic the ambivalent complicity of parents and the comparative absence of people diagnosed with some form of autism[2] in ASD research, treatment, and advocacy organizations; this we take together with the uniform character of assistance offered by government agencies and schools.

Following from the problematic, we focus on parents' everyday actions, and how they generalize and abstract their children's identities and lives, through the diagnosis and "access to assistance" process. Specifically, we map parents' navigation of ASD services, treatments, and interventions, and examine how these relationships effectively silence the experiences of people diagnosed with ASD, and instead objectify it as both an enemy and a business opportunity. Finally, we look at how ASD spectrumization relates to and serves the larger processes of financialization and austerity.

ASD PARENTS AND CHILDREN

Sofia's experience with ASD began when her son David was diagnosed not long after starting public school. Since receiving this diagnosis, states Sofia, she began to reinterpret both of her sons' "behaviors" as infants, and even in the womb, as indicators of autism. "Classic signs" and "behaviors" included "head-banging" and "rocking back and forth" in their cribs. Even Anthony's speech difficulties, because of a severe tongue injury, were linked to autism—his bitten tongue was attributed to "uncoordinated body movements" associated with autism.

When David and Anthony started school a month late, they encountered problems. Sofia describes their teachers as not "supportive" or "tolerant" of their shyness and their desire to work closely together "as a unit." Teachers decided it was "healthier" to break up "the unit," so David was placed in a Kindergarten Intervention Program at a different school where he was given extra attention by educational assistants. Sofia explained that there were a number of social factors that led to this placement. According to Sofia, their late start at school was related to the unwelcoming attitude of the teachers. She also recounts the feeling of being an isolated, young, working-class, Eastern European immigrant woman in a predominantly "Anglo-Saxon neighborhood" and being blamed for her children's difficulties adjusting to kindergarten. She says: "It was a very negative environment ... and there was animosity towards the children [and herself] immediately." In a situation where her entire family felt out of place and unwelcome, the special attention and services associated with an Asperger's diagnosis were warmly welcomed.[3]

Soon, through a process that "wasn't very clear," a doctor became heavily involved in the boys' lives, regularly assessing their development. Sofia felt that this involvement contributed very little to the twins' lives. Both of her children also had Individual Education Plans (IEPs) that were updated regularly until the time they graduated from high school. These IEPs continually galvanized the autism diagnosis and framed the most intimate details of their lives—their relationships with other students, the academic interests they were able to pursue, and the ways in which their behavior and performance were understood. When Sofia and her first husband were in the midst of a difficult divorce, David went to live part time with his father and grandparents.

During this time, he was heavily medicated with Ritalin, "because it made life easier" for the father and teachers when David "acted out." According to Sofia, David called his years on Ritalin "the lost years" because he remembers very little from that time. Later on, Anthony was also given Ritalin; however, he became physically ill from the drug and was quickly taken off of it. Both boys are now pursuing post-secondary education and being diagnosed again using the new DSM-5 to improve their educational accommodations for autism.

The many revisions to the way autism has been conceptualized in the DSM (discussed later in the chapter) were not discussed in detail during the interview. What became clear, however, was that getting support for her sons' school difficulties hinged on their attaining "status" through the DSM. Unlike many of the parents described in the ASD literature (in particular, see Gruson-Wood 2014; McGuire 2015), Sofia is not involved with autism advocacy. Nevertheless, she is involved in organizing her sons' lives, taking particular pride in her role in helping them attain higher education. She organizes their records, helps them with their homework, and counsels them in all decision making.

As an immigrant, working-class parent, Sofia has been very isolated. Trying to support her sons was a process of "trial and error." She had little access to resources and information, especially in comparison to the well-to-do parents that appear to be more actively engaged in the autism advocacy described by McGuire (2016). Sofia was not familiar with prominent autism advocacy organizations such as "Autism Speaks"; nor did she know very much about leading autism treatments such as Applied Behavioral Analysis (ABA) and Intensive Behavioral Intervention (IBI).

Autism and the DSM

Sofia's experiences raising her children have been highly structured by the texts, metaphors, and medical narratives of the autism spectrum. To understand the current configuration of ASD, it is necessary to have an understanding of the historical evolution of autism, as reflected in the ever-changing DSM. Autism as a concept was first articulated by Leo Kanner in 1943; however, the DSM did not include autism as a psychiatric diagnosis until the DSM-III edition in 1980. It appeared under the new category of Pervasive Development Disorders, which distinguished autism for the first time as a diagnosis different from Mental Retardation and separated it, for the first time since DSM-I, from Childhood Schizophrenia.

By the release of DSM-IV in 1994, Pervasive Development Disorders had expanded to include five discrete diagnostic entities: Autistic Disorder, Rett Disorder, Childhood Disintegrative Disorder, Asperger's Disorder, and Pervasive Development Disorder Not Otherwise Specified. These five entities were described as qualitatively different from each other. Rett Disorder was removed from the DSM-5 when its genetic basis was "discovered," and the remaining four Pervasive Development Disorders were incorporated under one diagnostic umbrella: Autism Spectrum Disorder. The new spectrum was rationalized by the American Psychiatric Association as "a scientific consensus that four previously separate disorders are actually a single condition with different levels of symptom severity in two core domains ... 1) deficits in social communication and social interaction and 2) restricted repetitive behaviors, interests, and activities" (DSM-5 Diagnostic Criteria, American Psychiatric Association 2013).[4]

For children diagnosed with ASD and their parents, the DSM subsequently has had a profound influence on everyday activities. It is what Burstow (2015) calls a "boss text, [texts] ... higher up in the hierarchy that influence both the creation and the deployment of other texts" (p. 18). It is important to note that the dramatic changes that autism has undergone via the DSM are not unique and are by no means based on scientific discovery. In *Psychiatry and the Business of Madness*, Bonnie Burstow (2015) argues that science is peripheral to these revisions. By examining the political and ideological motivations for the changes, Burstow demonstrates how "dramatic ongoing changes are a 'given.' Research, such as it is, is not the driving force of change but rather the justification or rationale" (p. 74).

As we traced the social relations of ASD, we found numerous examples of this. For instance, the DSM-5 was conceived a priori as being a project of "dimensionalizing" all mental disorders. Whooley (2014) recounts that the DSM-5 task force envisioned it as a new model for diagnosis, changing the conception of mental disorders from that of *"qualitatively* distinct from mental health" to that of a matter of degree: Mental illness would be reconceived as *"quantitatively* different" than mental health "through the introduction of scales; a difference of magnitude, not in kind" (italics in original). The attempt was to place "well-being" and "mental disorders" on a spectrum by providing numerical severity scales for each diagnosis. Perhaps not surprisingly, this proved too difficult for most diagnoses. Except in the case of a psychosis severity scale and the spectrumization of the former Pervasive Development Disorders under ASD, the dimensionalizing DSM-5 diagnosis was abandoned.

Parents and the DSM

Parents have been vocal advocates and fundamental to the research and treatment of autism since the wave of deinstitutionalization in North America during the 1960s. As parents more frequently cared for their children at home, their interest in developing customized cures and treatments grew. They sought explanations and treatments and in the process built new therapeutic alliances with researchers, occupational therapists, educators, and activists. This blurred the connection between lay and expert knowledge (Eyal 2013, p. 868) and often positioned parents as partners in the diagnosis and treatment of their children. However, not all parents participated equally in such partnerships. Mothers, in particular, were blamed for their children's "conditions." A diagnosis of autism also had class and racial characteristics.

Access to a diagnosis remained reserved for children of white, bourgeois women, who were called "refrigerator mothers."[5] It was these women who rejected the patriarchal ideologies embedded within psychiatric theories and practices during that time. They sought to be "good mother nurturers" (McGuire 2016) who championed fundraising efforts and advocacy campaigns. Conversely, Getfield (2015) describes how working-class immigrant mothers were framed as "disengaged" or "hard to reach" even as government policies impeded their access to supports and resources.

In DSM-III's section on "Predisposing factors" we can see the first evidence of parent advocacy with respect to the diagnostic criteria for autism; it states: "In the past, certain familial interpersonal factors were thought to predispose to the development of this syndrome, but recent studies do not support this view" (p. 89). Although not explicitly specified, this is almost certainly a response to the "refrigerator mother" thesis that had surrounded autism's etiology for decades.

Demanding a Spectrumized Diagnosis

The most recent diagnostic codification of ASD in the 2013 DSM revision appears to be motivated by practical desires for ease of diagnosis and popular support for access to resources. Numerous researchers have pointed out that the autism diagnosis is closely associated with critical forms of social support (Blumberg et al. 2013; Eyal 2013). Advocacy groups pushed for a spectrum diagnosis in part because categorical conceptions of Pervasive Development Disorders sometimes made it difficult to access services for "higher-functioning" individuals and their families. Effectively lumping all Pervasive Development Disorders into a single "spectrum" could allow clinicians to tailor diagnoses to suit local criteria for service delivery (Ne'eman 2010). In this way lobbying for the spectrumization of ASD often was motivated by parents' socioeconomic demands.

Such socioeconomic demands are shaped by widespread austere structural changes to public education, research, and medicine. As we drew on Sofia's and our own lived, everyday experiences, we came to understand how parents, teachers, and care providers mediate and reproduce the ruling relations of austerity in their everyday actions with the public education and medical bureaucracies in Canada. Like many working-class immigrant mothers (Getfield 2015), Sofia found it difficult to do the navigating necessary to secure public resources for her sons, David and Anthony. It became very clear in our interview that getting a diagnosis was the linchpin for accessing much-needed "assistance" or support and resources. She told us that when David was diagnosed with Asperger's Syndrome, "suddenly there was help available."

Sofia explained that, rather than being framed as a "troubled child," David was theorized as a child with a "social impairment [and] probably other physiological issues." Ultimately, she felt that this diagnosis made it possible to access a more supportive environment for him, stating that "it would be better for [David] if he gets into [a school] environment where they want [him], over being in an environment where they can't stand him. It was simple as that." That help had been denied without an official diagnosis was clearly demonstrated by Anthony's experience; he was diagnosed years later than David. "Lacking" a diagnosis, Anthony was more regularly shunned and alienated in school when he was slow at catching on or behaved "abnormally."

Sofia's experience of having a diagnosis become a gateway for much-needed health and education supports for her children is not surprising, given that without one, little support was available. To obtain a diagnosis, of course, one must move through the channels shown in Figure 5.1, activating the pertinent DSM criteria. This activity closely links the parents' and children's life experiences and relationship with the primary "boss text" of psychiatry.

Two specific characteristics of the DSM become particularly relevant for this investigation: (1) its changeability, as it surges through various ideological revisions; and (2) its power to dehumanize and alienate the experiences of people with DSM diagnoses. The latter is such that their diagnosis comes to dominate one's identity and to explain almost all aspects of behavior, thereby obscuring and negating historical, social, political, and economic dimensions of the diagnosed person.

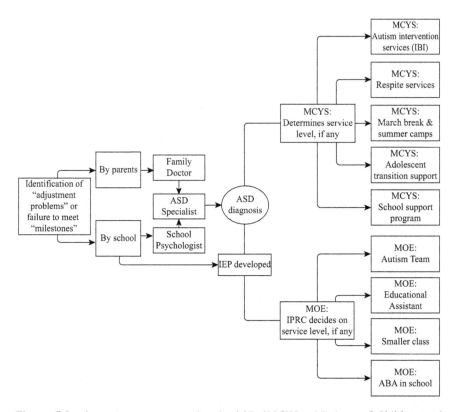

Figure 5.1 Access to support services in ASD (MCYS – Ministry of Children and Youth Service, MOE – Ministry of Education, IBI – Intensive Behavioural Intervention, IPRC – Identification, Placement and Review Committee, ABA – Applied Behavioral Analysis)

Accessing "Assistance"

Accessing free or subsidized "assistance" for a child experiencing problems, as already noted, is extremely difficult without a psychiatric diagnosis. Figure 5.1 shows this process. In Ontario, the identification of "adjustment," "language," or "milestone" problems may be identified by either a parent or by the child's school, but "professional advice" and an official diagnosis must be obtained before access to assistance is granted. This begins with a family doctor referral to an ASD specialist. Specialists use DSM-based diagnostic questionnaires, checklists, and other such texts to make or exclude a diagnosis of ASD.

When a diagnosis of ASD is made, activation of the DSM text begins for parents, as they learn a new language and begin to negotiate the world of autism services and care. Parents must think and act within the world of ASD in order to serve their child's needs because no other service avenue exists. In effect, the DSM as a "boss text" activates the relations of ruling for both parents and children diagnosed with ASD, "capturing" them and narrowing their ideological and material scope of survival strategies and alternatives. Social and historical dimensions of the child's behavior become "accounted for" through the diagnosis.

A diagnosis opens up avenues for "assistance" that, while usually limited to the pathologized scope of the DSM, nevertheless assist families who are struggling to care for their children. Assistance can take the form of "treatment," such as behavioral interventions or drugs, funding, specialized attention, and educational planning, or "respite." In Ontario, assistance for ASD is primarily through the Ministry of Children and Youth Services and the Ministry of Education. Both pathways are activated through a report, signed by an authorized medical professional, certifying that a diagnosis of ASD has been made. Through the DSM-5, a "severity value" of 1–3 is also available, registering degree of "impairment" for "Social communication" and "Restricted, repetitive behaviors," thereby indicating numerically where each diagnosed person sits "on the spectrum" (DSM-5 Diagnostic Criteria 2015, pp. 50–55).

A diagnosis of ASD does not automatically lead to assistance, but it does permit access to a second level of assessment (Programs and Services for Children with Autism, n.d.), whereby children with an ASD diagnosis are screened for program eligibility. Access to information, "respite services," therapies, and school transition support is available if the diagnosis is "toward the severe end of the autism spectrum" (see http://www.children.gov.on.ca/htdocs/English/specialneeds/autism/programs.aspx). Families who are refused service based on the Ministry's criteria are advised to "request an independent review of that decision" (see http://www.children.gov.on.ca/htdocs/English/specialneeds/autism/programs.aspx). All this being the case, even families whose child receives an ASD diagnosis may have to fight with the Ministry for access to assistance on grounds of having a "severe enough" case. The DSM therefore is activated by parents even when care is denied.

Children who receive access to assistance through the Ministry of Children and Youth Services are given IBI—an intensive (3–5 days/week) form of ABA. These interventions use principles of learning theory and behaviorism to increase "desirable behaviors" and extinguish "undesirable" ones. In Ontario, wait times for this type of support may be as long as two to three years (Gordon, 2015).

When a child diagnosed with ASD reaches school age, the Ministry of Education becomes the primary gatekeeper for services. The Ministry of Children and Youth Services provides support to school boards through ASD consultants, who work with schools in order to provide service. After receipt of a medical report indicating an ASD diagnosis, a consultation with educators, parents, and involved professionals (e.g., psychologist, social worker, ASD team members) is convened at what is called an Identification, Placement, and Review Committee meeting. This meeting has a particular format and uses "eduspeak" (i.e., language and acronyms used by educators), which may be confusing for parents, but nevertheless uses the child's ASD diagnosis to determine service level and the most "appropriate" setting for the child at school. An IEP, described by Sofia in our interview, is developed for the child in order to record specialized "needs" and placement details.

The Individual Education Plan is a legal document that compels educators to comply with the text, magnifying the DSM text's capacity to "rule" by providing access to support only through its representations. Policy/Program Memorandum 140 (Programs and Services for Children with Autism, n.d.), released by the Ministry of Education in 2006, also compels teachers and educational assistants to use ABA principles in their work with students who have an ASD diagnosis. As a result of their identification through the Identification, Placement, and Review Committee process, students with a diagnosis of ASD may receive placement in a smaller class; have an educational assistant who works with them some, or all, of the time; and have access to School Board/Ministry of Children and Youth Services ASD support team consultation. At all levels of the process, parents can only access care and support through their child's diagnosis and the texts that diagnosis has generated, thereby leading them to continually activate the DSM.

Bringing Out New DSMs

As shown in Figure 5.2, the experiences of those diagnosed with ASD and their parents are captive within the DSM creation process. Before a new DSM is released, work groups periodically release proposed changes to academics so that they can be studied according to medicalized protocols. Such studies provide not only feedback to work groups but also function as validation for the DSM to come. When a new version of the DSM is released, it triggers a cascade of responses within academia, including the development of rating scales, diagnostic tools, and manuals, that set the stage for the creation of intellectual property related to diagnosis and treatment. Popular texts (e.g., articles and websites) share information but refer clients to medical professionals, who are the gateway for diagnosis, and therefore assistance.

ASD and the Current Capitalist Reality

When parents seek help for their children through medical personnel, schools, or government agencies, they activate the DSM through the tools and education associated with them. Capitalist processes are intertwined with this activation because of the proprietary nature of medical education, as well as diagnostic tools and services. Particularly in institutional clinical settings, technicians and paraprofessionals can administer simplified diagnostic clinical products, saving institutions money by minimizing their use of professionals. Hospitals, schools, and other government institutions involved in ASD are therefore not only subject to the pressures of capital accumulation through use of these proprietary texts but also are driven to use them to save money or fall in line with "austerity measures."

Commitments to austerity have led powerful institutions to begin limiting the ways in which they recognize the DSM as a boss text by creating their own texts that define criteria for service. For example, some Ontario School Boards have a higher threshold for the identification of a learning disability than does

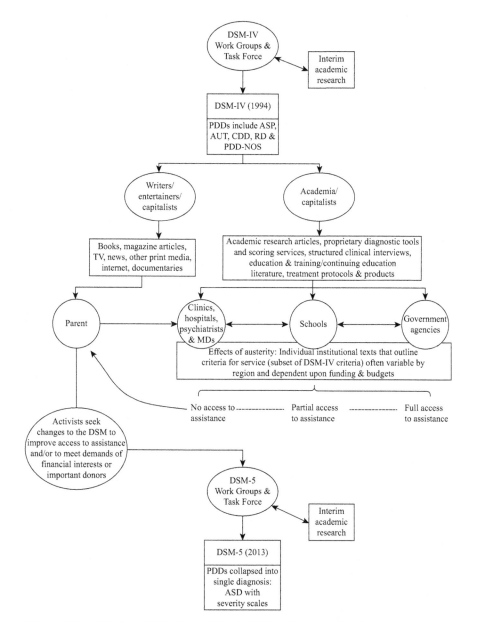

Figure 5.2 ASD from DSM-IV to DSM-5 (PDD – Pervasive Development Disorder, ASP – Asperger's, AUT – Autism, CDD – Childhood Disintegrative Disorder, RT – Rett Disorder, PDD-NOS – Pervasive Development Disorder Not Otherwise Specified)

the Ontario College of Psychologists. This means that even when a community psychologist diagnoses a student with a learning disability, the school board may not officially recognize it as such. Even though this may not limit access to school-based assistance, it opens up space for changes to the way that schools are funded for this assistance, by, for example, changing teacher–student ratios for special education services and effectively passing the obligation to provide services on to schools (Devji 2014). With respect to ASD in Ontario, this same process is at work. The Ministry of Children and Youth Services only provides access to services if a child has a "severe enough" diagnosis.

For parents who have been denied service or who have experienced long wait times, institutional texts that limit access to care are perceived as creating great harm. Parents are immersed in the language of the DSM and receive nearly all of their information from texts that are informed by it. As Figure 5.2 illustrated earlier, parents who are refused or have inadequate assistance remain captive within the DSM text. Rather than pursuing a broader vision of how assistance can be accessed and by whom, assistance remains pinned to the diagnosis of ASD. Thus, parents often focus on changing the diagnosis, rather than other structural changes.

Working-class parents, in particular, have turned to (capitalist) advocacy groups and allowed them to speak on their behalf, operating within the DSM conception of ASD, rather than seeking alternatives to the system. Such advocacy groups have worked with the professional community and the DSM-5 work group to create a simplified and noncategorical conception of autism and related disorders. It remains to be seen how this will impact "care" in the future. Still, the DSM-5 provides clear benefits to intellectual property capitalists. Because spectrumization renders "ASD severity" measurable, individual changes in severity can be tracked over time by proprietary technician-administered diagnostic tools. Interventions can be aimed at reducing symptom severity, and the "evidence" for treatment protocols can be evaluated for "efficacy" and marketed accordingly.

The objectification of "ASD symptoms" creates opportunities for products to emerge that may reduce what is seen as symptom severity but do not necessarily improve quality of life. More subtly, however, the reduction of ASD to a generic measurable spectrum creates a greater subjective need on the part of parents to have their child's particular needs understood. Because deficits in public funding create greater gaps and discontinuities in service delivery and exacerbate class divisions among parents, the DSM-5 simultaneously creates a greater requirement on the part of parents to communicate their particular child's needs. Together, these circumstances create the conditions for the development of private service delivery resources of all types. Also, because "the spectrum" in DSM-5's autism spectrum disorder presents a potential blurring with normalcy, lay- and self-"diagnosis" become possible in ways that can present opportunities for capitalist "self-help" products.

Which brings us to the increasingly dominant role of financial markets in the process of capitalist accumulation.[6] Specifically, we examine briefly how the "capture" of ASD is shaped by the social relations of financializing ASD advocacy, shrinking public education resources, and rapidly eroding the Canadian healthcare and welfare state.

Austerity and Financialization

Over the last three decades, globalized financial restructuring has intensified, aggressively undermining the Keynesian welfare model for healthcare, disability, and income support in Canada. Taxes on corporate profits have been halved, federally from 28 % in 2000 to 15 % in 2015, and provincially in Ontario during this timeframe from 14 % to 8 %, reducing government income (Sanger 2014), which in turn has rationalized austerity. At the same time, public institutions like schools and hospitals have been increasingly configured as isolated entities that are subject to rules of accounting that portray them not as public goods but as costs (Miller and Power 2013). These changes are part of what is called "neoliberal restructuring," which ideologically reshapes state health and education provision into "markets best handled by the private sector" in order to manage costs and produce profit (see Harvey 2005).

In this context, healthcare and disability services have been restructured through public–private partnerships (P3s) and financial investments. In Ontario, this has increasingly deprived disabled people of social services and welfare provision (Hande and Kelly 2015) because public goods are reenvisioned as both the responsibility of individuals and sites of private profit-making. Meanwhile, health insurance, healthcare institutions (Whiteside 2009), research facilities (see McGuire 2016), patented pharmaceutical and therapeutic interventions, diagnostic measures, and technological innovations (Grand Challenges Canada 2013) are turned into hugely profitable financial markets (Hande 2014).

Heather Whiteside (2009, 2011) discusses the increasing role of public–private partnership funding models as key mechanisms for the achievement of this neoliberal financial restructuring. P3s typically involve private enterprises (e.g., architectural firms, financial institutions, construction companies, and maintenance firms) partnering with public ones; that is, bidding on provincial projects and using public funds to execute them. With multiple P3s disasters in Canada (see Boase 2000), Whiteside (2009, 2011) argues that the benefits of the models are mostly ideological. In reality, they facilitate the piecemeal conversion of public sector into private investments that contractually guarantee future revenue streams.

Public–private partnerships are a softer, gradual form of privatization that are implemented in politically sensitive areas such as education and healthcare (Whiteside 2009). In Canada, there are harbingers of P3s in ASD service provision in Ontario (discussed later in this chapter) and in higher education.[7] In this context, marginalized immigrant parents and medicalized children, such as Sofia and her twin sons, that are "starved through austerity" (Magnusson 2013, p. 76) understandably welcome the opportunities provided by research and therapeutic initiatives even if they are motivated by private financial interests. Autism spectrum disorder research and advocacy organizations, such as "Autism Speaks" and "Spectrum of Hope," reveal a maze of P3s and private financial interests and investments, particularly in the US context.

These processes of privatization and austerity have implications for how disability and psychiatric diagnoses are treated. Kelly Fritsch (2015) argues that, in this context, the narrative of cure may be activated, but nevertheless, the "cure is an intervention that only occurs once and thus is limited in the scope of its potential profitability" (p. 27). Instead, lifelong interventions (e.g., behavioral therapies and supports) are much more profitable. The welfare state has become supplanted by a highly financialized disability industry wherein binary concepts of healthy/unhealthy and normality/abnormality were reorganized as spectrums, as in the case of ASD.

These gradations and spectrums open up financial markets and stimulate innovation for chronically necessary interventions (e.g., therapies and supplements) that enhance people's capacities. As Whiteside (2009) argues, this restructuring is because of a crisis of capital accumulation requiring the unravelling of the Keynsian welfare state. Arguably, these days "successful" autism advocacy organizations are those that are being "captured by market rationality" and are intertwined with forms of austerity and financialization.

The Business of ASD

According to Anne McGuire, "[n]o single organization exemplifies the lucrative intermingling of corporate interest and autism advocacy more clearly than 'Autism Speaks'" (2016, p. 128). Its board of directors is composed of leaders in financial investment and management, many of whom have children labeled ASD (see autismspeaks.org/about-us/board-directors). Having the financial clout to dictate the direction of autism research, therapies, services, and interventions effectively, "Autism Speaks" has become both a leader in government policy and financial investment, a model for autism advocacy and a lightning rod for criticism from the autistic community (see "Ask an Autistic" 2014; autisticadvocacy.org). Indeed, few autism organizations, in either Canada or the United States, are without an explicit link with "Autism Speaks." As McGuire so compellingly argues, the report has led the way in branding autism for consumers, while also inextricably relating autism research and treatment priorities to the financial markets.

At the United Nations's inaugural World Autism Awareness Day, "Autism Speaks" honored the event by ringing the New York Stock Exchange morning bell, symbolically signaling that "hope" for people diagnosed with ASD must be linked with financial trading. Even when the markets sank in 2007, "investment" in ASD remained a key priority. When in 2009, the US government passed the "American Recovery and Reinvestment Act" to "stimulate the economy," nearly $100 million was earmarked for autism research, particularly in the areas of biomedical and biotechnical investigations. This, coupled with the millions in government investment through the US "Combating Autism

Act," has meant big business for ASD advocacy organizations and has attracted hosts of, what McGuire (2016) describes as, "philanthrocapitalists" to the booming financial world of autism.

In Canada, the financialization of ASD is much less developed; however, as the discourse around an "autism epidemic" and the enthusiasm for the notion of "spectrums" grows, the incentive for new research, treatments, and products increases. Because research shows that parents of children diagnosed with ASD do not necessarily choose treatment options based on efficacy (Miller et al. 2011), but instead on factors, such as time commitment or ease of implementation (Green 2007), there is potential for highly exploitative or even fraudulent private ASD services to emerge.

With diagnoses of autism-spectrum disorders increasing (Matson and Kozlowski 2011), market analysts call autism spectrum disorder a "chronically underserved market" (Opportunity Analyzer 2014). It remains to be seen how this market will be "served," by whom, and to what effect. ASD exists in a space where "markets" have only begun to emerge. Because it is new, the spectrumization of ASD leaves so-called "market construction" open for creation. With respect to the *business* of ASD, new lines of reasoning and categorization may be financially useful—particularly as the public sphere is increasingly restructured—opening up space for private interests to serve these emergent "markets" and "add value" to dwindling public resources.

It is incredibly important to emphasize here the multiple and disturbing threats these forms of financialized advocacy and services pose for people diagnosed with ASD. As parents take over the leadership roles in organizations, they effectively remove the voices, experiences, and self-described interests of those diagnosed with ASD. These processes are interrelated with the relations of dispossession, austerity, and pathologization, as described by Fritsch (2015), Hande and Kelly (2015), and Whiteside (2009, 2011). Anne McGuire (2016) describes at length how organizations like "Autism Speaks" reproduce frames of combat and eradication in their work around autism. In worst-case scenarios, both the ASD diagnostic criteria and the ideological frames coming from eugenics and war are activated to justify parents' murder of children diagnosed with autism.

Members of the autistic community sometimes object to the research and services funded through these kinds of advocacy groups. For example, although many standard treatments, such as ABA, are popular among parents, Julia Gruson-Wood (2014) has pointed out that autistic children who have undergone these therapies often grow up to be vocal opponents of them—sometimes likening them to abuse. The Autistic Self Advocacy Network, a disability rights group led by people diagnosed with autism, also has condemned the use of aversive interventions (e.g., pain or electroshock) as part of Applied Behavior Analysis (Autistic Self Advocacy Network 2014a, 2015). The voices from within the autistic community have been ignored by work groups revising the DSM and the myriad related "treatment protocols" that have been devised. Instead, even in Canadian universities, such as York University, we are beginning to see increasing development of ABA interventions in the private sector and directly marketed to parents.[8]

ASD Philanthrocapitalism in Canada

Albeit the financialization of ASD is not nearly as advanced in Canada as in the USA, yet the framework is being laid. In Ontario, both the New Haven Learning Centre and the Spectrum of Hope proposed Kae Martin Campus as having positioned themselves as exciting new "resources" for parents with children diagnosed with autism spectrum disorder. Framed as sites of researched pedagogies, therapies, and interventions for ASD, the private financial interests in these institutions are often overlooked or invisible. Gruson-Wood's research (2013) on the Kae Martin Campus inspired us to look closer at this proposed project as an important Ontario-based example of the emerging forms of ASD services and initiatives.

The Spectrum of Hope Foundation was formed in 2011 to raise funds for the Kae Martin Campus, which is intended to be a "regional education facility that integrates best practices in health and wellness and applied research into its educational programming" (spectrumofhope.ca/foundation/, n.d.). Similar to the US "Autism Speaks" model of philanthrocapitalist advocacy, Spectrum of Hope's board represents significant financial interests (e.g., Treelawn Investment Corp., Alamos Gold, and Element Financial Corporation), with a smattering of representation from parents of children diagnosed with ASD. The proposed Kae Martin Campus is premised as a P3s that will "add value to an existing service network" (Spectrum of Hope Foundation, Autism 2015).

York University also plays an important role. An adjunct faculty member is already on Spectrum of Hope's payroll at Kae Martin Campus's Early Intervention and Preschool Program. In turn, Spectrum of Hope provides critical funding for York University's ASD research initiatives. Part of this funding is used in its Asperger Mentoring Program (n.d.), which allows graduate students not only to support but also conduct research on "autistic mentees" in order to "apply" and hone their research skills. As Sofia explained to us during her interview, the very existence of this program lures parents to enroll their ASD-labeled adult children in York University.

The York University focus on ASD seems to be a key site for meshing public and private interests into research and therapeutic initiatives for people diagnosed with ASD. In 2012, York's autism research chair was granted $2 million to study the relationship between autism and bullying. A large portion of this funding was provided by organizations with significant financial interests, including "Autism Speaks" and The Sinneave Family Foundation (2015)—with York University matching the funding that these organizations were to provide (Allen 2012).

These partnerships "capture" parents in unexpected ways. Sofia repeatedly mentioned to us how David receives the best accommodation and service support he has ever received throughout his schooling in higher education.

Even though Sofia and her sons may not be aware of the ruling relationship structuring and coordinating these research and therapeutic agendas, she knows that the programs are the best of the limited resources available to help her son navigate a university. The stress and ambivalence of these relations for parents has been examined by a number of researchers (e.g., see Hastings and Johnson 2001; Wagner 2010; Buescher et al. 2014); still the experiences of autistic youth remain relatively underresearched.

Nevertheless, autistic social movements are ramping up politically. Organizations, such as the Association for Autistic Community, the Autistic Self Advocacy Network, and the Autism Women's Network, are finding their way into the political limelight and are exposing the financialization of ASD. How these organizations frame and address the financialization of autism spectrum disorder, if at all, is also underresearched; therefore we hope this chapter weaves these connections in a way that is realistically useful for activists diagnosed with ASD.

Concluding Remarks

For working-class parents like Sofia, abstract ASD language and diagnostic criteria capture and dominate life so that options and trajectories for material resources, such as education and healthcare, appear unavoidably tied up with a diagnosis. What is often hidden and obscured from the day-to-day activities of accessing this assistance and the resources are the complex, multileveled ruling relationships that structure them. By mapping ASD research, services, and resources, we have begun to reveal larger relations of austerity, philanthrocapitalism, and financialization.

Furthermore, and perhaps most important, now we better understand how these ruling relations come to directly act on parents and children labeled with ASD, *and* how parents, in particular, become active, if unwitting, agents in reproducing these relationships every time they activate an ASD text or narrative in the process of caring for their children. We hope that the activities and relations we have mapped here demonstrate how these shifts in ASD diagnosis and treatment are more than discursive or cultural. These social relations also are structured by working-class parents' material motivations for healthcare and education resources made scarce by mushrooming global financialization. These social relationships are actively (re)produced by white bourgeois parents interested in the financialization of ASD advocacy, research, and treatment options.

Through the analysis in this chapter we expose and begin to understand the dangerous and violent implications of social, scientific, diagnostic, and financialized processes that silence the experiences and material interests of children diagnosed with ASD. Hopefully, this analysis will be helpful for children and adults whose interests are being "overruled." As Dorothy Smith (2005) states, "knowing how things work, how they're put together, is invaluable for those who often have to struggle in the dark" (p. 32).

NOTES

1. All participants' names are pseudonyms.
2. From here on, ASD refers to DSM-5's Autism Spectrum Disorder, but it is important to note that some people have not been officially diagnosed with ASD, even if they have been diagnosed with one of the DSM-IV PDDs. In addition, some people reject DSM-5's ASD outright, identifying with DSM-IV's separate categories (i.e., Asperger's or autism). In this chapter we use the terminology that seems most appropriate for the given context.
3. This is consistent with Getfield's (2015) analysis of working-class immigrant parents with children diagnosed with learning disabilities or mental illness.
4. Prior to DSM-5, autism was sometimes conceptualized as a spectrum, but only metaphorically. Anne McGuire (2016) explains that the 1979 Camberwell Study conceptualized autism as a "spectrum disorder" that arranged a variety of "deficits," "syndromes," and "disorders" on a scale of "mild" to "severe."
5. The "refrigerator mother" hypothesis of autism was first presented by Austrian-American therapist Bruno Bettelheim, who expounded on the idea in his book, *The Empty Fortress* (1967). Influenced by psychoanalysis, citing the results of experiments on infant monkeys that had been removed from their mothers (Deisinger 2011), and comparing autistic children to concentration camp survivors (Raz 2014), Bettelheim asserted that autism was caused by emotionally distant, inattentive, and cold mothers (Verhoeff 2013). Despite the fact that there was no evidence to support this highly gendered and misogynist explanation, it persisted for many years. Such woman-blaming persists in theories of autism, from mother's choices about diet, medical care, lifestyle, and partner choices (Walden 2012).
6. See Magnusson (2015) for a detailed historical account of this process.
7. In the realm of higher education, Jamie Magnusson (2013) describes how "[t]he austerity policy environment encourages claw backs in public funding to education and community infrastructure at the same time that a surplus is accumulating … and being invested into infrastructures of incarceration and militarism" (p. 76).
8. See, for example, one of York University's signature autism research initiatives, Secret Agents Society (n.d.)—see http://ddmh.lab.yorku.ca/secret-agents-society/. This initiative is funded in large part through a partnership with Spectrum of Hope, a Canadian ASD advocacy organization modeled on the "Autism Speaks" philanthrocapitalist-styled advocacy.

REFERENCES

Allen, K. (2012, November 4). The autism project: Autism research chair will look at bullying. *The Toronto Star*. Retrieved from http://www.thestar.com/news/investigations/2012/11/04/the_autism_project_autism_research_chair_will_look_at_bullying.html

American Psychiatric Association. (2013). *Highlights of changes from DSM-IV-TR to DSM-5*. Retrieved July 3 from http://www.dsm5.org/Documents/Autism%20Spectrum%20Disorder%20Fact%20Sheet.pdf.

Ask an autistic—What's wrong with Autism Speaks?. (2014, March 13). *Youtube*. Retrieved July 7, 2015, from https://www.youtube.com/watch?v=ez936r2F35U

Asperger Mentoring Program (AMP). (n.d.). *Children's learning projects*. Retrieved July 7, 2015, from https://bebko.apps01.yorku.ca/clp/?page_id=132

Autistic Self Advocacy Network. (n.d.). *Nothing about us without us.* Retrieved July 7, 2015, from http://autisticadvocacy.org/

Autistic Self Advocacy Network. (2014a). *ASAN letter: California should cover more than ABA.* Retrieved July 19, 2015, from http://autisticadvocacy.org/2014/10/asan-letter-california-should-cover-more-than-aba/

Autistic Self Advocacy Network. (2014b). *Joint letter to the sponsors of Autism Speaks.* Retrieved July 19, 2015, from http://autisticadvocacy.org/2014/01/2013-joint-letter-to-the-sponsors-of-autism-speaks/

Autistic Self Advocacy Network. (2015). *ASAN statement on JRC at Association for Behavior Analysis International conference.* Retrieved July 19, 2015, from http://autisticadvocacy.org/2015/05/asan-statement-on-jrc-at-association-for-behavior-analysis-international-conference/

Bettelheim, B. (1967). *The empty fortress.* New York: The Free Press.

Blumberg, S. J., Bramlett, M. D., Kogan, M. D., et al. (2013). Changes in prevalence of parent-reported Autism Spectrum Disorder in school-aged U.S. children: 2007 to 2011-2012. *National Health Statistics Report, 65,* 1-11.

Boase, J. P. (2000). Beyond government? The appeal of public-private partnerships. *Canadian Public Administration, 43,* 75–92.

Buescher, A. V. S., Cidav, Z., Knapp, M., & Mandell, D. S. (2014). Costs of Autism Spectrum Disorders in the United Kingdom and the United States. *JAMA Pediatrics, 168,* 721–128.

Burstow, B. (2015). *Psychiatry and the business of madness: An ethical and epistemological accounting.* New York: Palgrave Macmillan.

Deisinger, J. A. (2011). History of Autism Spectrum Disorders. In A. F. Rotatori, F. E. Obiakor, & J. P. Bakken (Eds.), *History of special education* (pp. 237–267). Bingley: Emerald Group Publishing Limited.

Devji, S. (2014). *The intricacies of inclusive schooling.* Unpublished manuscript, Department of Educational Leadership and Policy Studies, Ontario Institute for Studies in Education, Toronto, ON.

Eyal, G. (2013). For a sociology of expertise: The social origins of the autism epidemic. *American Journal of Sociology, 118,* 863–907.

Fritsch, K. (2015). Gradations of debility and capacity: Biocapitalism and the neoliberalization of disability relations. *Canadian Journal of Disability Studies, 4*(2), 12–48.

Getfield, J. (2015, June). *Family engagement policy: Forging relationships that transform the other.* Paper presented at annual conference of the Canadian Disability Studies Association, University of Ottawa, Ottawa.

Gordon, A. (2015, April 17). Chronic wait times persist for families coping with autism. *The Toronto Star.* Retrieved from http://www.thestar.com/life/2015/04/17/chronic-wait-times-persist-for-families-coping-with-autism.html

Grand Challenges Canada. (2013, November 21). *Imaginative: 83 bold innovations to improve global health receive grand challenges Canada funding.* Retrieved December 6, 2015, from http://www.grandchallenges.ca/wp-content/uploads/StarsinGlobalHealth-Round5-NewsRelease-Nov2013-EN.pdf.

Green, V. A. (2007). Parental experience with treatments for autism. *Journal of Developmental and Physical Disabilities, 19,* 91–101.

Gruson-Wood, J. (2013, June). *The edge of hybrid spaces: Autistic youth and the home-lab.* Paper presented at the annual conference at Canadian Disability Studies Association Conference. Victoria: University of Victoria.

Gruson-Wood, J. (2014). *Investigating the everyday practice of evidence-based behavioural therapies.* Presentation for Healthcare, Technology and Place: CIHR Strategic Research and Training. Retrieved July 3, 2015, from https://www.kaltura.com/index.php/extwidget/preview/partner_id/1499521/uiconf_id/16451821/entry_id/1_kalpaa5n/embed/auto?&flashvars%5BstreamerType%5D=auto

Hande, M. J. (2014, May). *Challenging the financialization of healthcare and disability through "commoning."* Paper presented at annual conference of the Society for Socialist Studies, St. Catherines: Brock University.

Hande, M. J., & Kelly, C. (2015). Organizing survival and resistance in austere times: Shifting disability activism and care politics in Ontario, Canada. *Disability & Society, 30*(7), 961–975.

Harvey, D. (2005). *A brief history of neoliberalism.* New York/Oxford: Oxford University Press.

Hastings, R. P., & Johnson, E. (2001). Stress in UK families conducting home-based behavioral intervention for the their young child with autism. *Journal of Autism and Developmental Disorders, 31*, 327–336.

Magnusson, J. (2013). Precarious learning and labour in financialized time. *Brock Education, 22*, 69–83.

Magnusson, J. (2015). Financialisation. In S. Mojab (Ed.), *Marxism and feminism* (pp. 142–162). London: Zed Books.

Matson, J. L., & Kozlowski, A. M. (2011). The increasing prevalence of autism spectrum disorders. *Research in Autism Spectrum Disorders, 5*, 418–425.

McGuire, A. (2015). Life worth defending: Bio-political frames of terror in the war on autism. In S. Tremain (Ed.), *Foucault and the government of disability* (2nd ed., pp. 350–371). Ann Arbor: University of Michigan Press.

McGuire, A. (2016). *The war on autism: On normative violence and the cultural production of autism advocacy.* Ann Arbor: University of Michigan Press.

Miller, P., & Power, M. (2013). Accounting, organizing, and economizing: Connecting accounting research and organization theory. *The Academy of Management Annals, 7*(1), 557–605. doi:10.1080/19416520.2013.783668

Miller, V. A., Schreck, K. A., Mulick, J. A., & Butter, E. (2011). Factors related to parents' choices of treatments for their children with Autism Spectrum Disorders. *Research in Autism Spectrum Disorders, 6*, 87–95.

Ne'eman, A. (2010). The future (and the past) of autism advocacy, or why the ASA's magazine, the advocate, wouldn't publish this piece. *Disability Studies Quarterly, 30.*

Ontario Ministry of Children and Youth Services. (2015). *Programs and services for children with autism: Who can receive autism intervention program services.* Retrieved July 3, 2015, from http://www.children.gov.on.ca/htdocs/English/topics/specialneeds/autism/programs.aspx

Opportunity Analyzer: Autism Spectrum Disorder—Opportunity Analysis and Forecasts to 2018. (2014). *ASD reports.* Retrieved July 3, 2015, from https://www.asdreports.com/market-research-report-101078/opportunityanalyzer-autism-spectrum-disorder-opportunity-analysis-forecasts

Raz, M. (2014). Deprived of touch: How maternal and sensory deprivation theory converged in shaping early debates over autism. *History of the Human Sciences, 27*(2), 75–96.

Sanger, T. (2014, September 19). Did corporate tax cuts really pay for themselves as Harper claims? *Huffington Post Canada.* Retrieved August 4, from http://www.huffingtonpost.ca/toby-sanger/corporate-tax-cuts_b_5844710.html

Secret Agent Society: Operation Regulation. (n.d.). *Developmental Disabilities and Mental Health Lab, York University.* Retrieved July 7, 2015, from http://ddmh.lab. yorku.ca/secret-agents-society

Secret Agent Society. Solving the Mystery of Social Encounters. (n.d.). *Social Skills Training Institute.* Retrieved June 3, 2015, from http://www.sst-institute.net.

The Sinneave Family Foundation. (2015). *Partners.* Retrieved July 7, 2015, from http://www.theabilityhub.org/about/partners.

Smith, D. (2005). *Institutional ethnography: A sociology for people.* Landham: Altamira Press.

Spectrum of Hope, About Autism. (2015). *Spectrum of Hope Foundation.* Retrieved February 11, 2015, from http://spectrumofhope.org/

Verhoeff, B. (2013). Autism in flux: A history of the concept from Leo Kanner to DSM-5. *History of Psychiatry, 24*(4), 442–458.

Wagner, E. L. (2010). *The parent check-up (PCU): Needs analysis, program development, service engagement, and feasibility in the applied behavior analysis setting* (Doctoral dissertation). Retrieved from Proquest. (3421002).

Walden, R. (2012). Autism: Origins unknown, but women still get the blame. *The Women's Health Activist, 37*, 11.

Whiteside, H. (2009). Canada's health care crisis: Accumulation by dispossession and the neoliberal fix. *Studies in Political Economy, 84*, 79–100.

Whiteside, H. (2011). Unhealthy policy: The political economy of Canadian public-private partnership hospitals. *Health Sociology Review, 20*, 258–268.

Whooley, O. (2014). Nosological reflections: The failure of DSM-5, the emergence of RDoC, and the decontextualization of mental distress. *Society and Mental Health, 4*(2), 92–110.

CHAPTER 6

Interrogating the Rights Discourse and Knowledge-Making Regimes of the "Movement for Global Mental Health"

Sonya L. Jakubec and Janet M. Rankin

INTRODUCTION

The explication of an evolving scale-up of research for global "mental health"[1] (GMH) and development, with which the lead author has been involved in as a program manager, nurse educator, and researcher for nearly 20 years, became a multilayered study—"research about research"—to uncover a vast and complex social organization (Jakubec 2015). This study grew as she assisted an international nongovernmental organization (NGO) called the Right to Livelihood[2] in its efforts to gain research funds and to advance research interests in the growing "movement for global mental health" (mGMH). It was, however, the NGO's original research process—a participatory model of community consultation—that first captured our interest.

The organization was unique in how it engaged with people labeled as "mentally ill," their family and professional "caregivers," and other local workers in order to advance people's right to inclusion and livelihoods. The NGO attempted to demonstrate what it, and others, construed as successes by including first-person accounts of what was being presented as the success of its model. This was accomplished within institutional documents over the first several years of program implementation (NGO Annual Report 2003[3]).

S.L. Jakubec (✉)
School of Nursing and Midwifery, Faculty of Health, Community and Education, Mount Royal University, Calgary, AB, Canada
e-mail: SJakubec@mtroyal.ca

J.M. Rankin
Faculty of Nursing, University of Calgary, Calgary, AB, Canada

103
B. Burstow (ed.), *Psychiatry Interrogated*,
DOI 10.1007/978-3-319-41174-3_6

Not unlike many organizations seeking to access research and program funding to harness credibility to expand programming at new sites, however, the Right to Livelihood needed more formal "evidence" of its "success."

In this chapter we attend to how this "evidence" came to be organized and to the various kinds of "mental health and development" knowledge that were being coordinated across healthcare and development sectors in Canada and globally. By different "mental health and development knowledge" we are referring to the various ways mental health and development were understood by workers at the NGO. Here we describe the knowledge of a variety of individuals who all find themselves oriented quite differently to particular kinds of health rights work. Researchers or program managers with an international NGO, a project manager with an official international development research organization, and someone doing grassroots advocacy are all workers for "mental health rights" who interact with and produce diverse kinds of (and differently authorized) knowledge.

Assisting the NGO in a research study on its model of "mental health and development," the lead author first experienced the point of rupture that is at the root of this study. She began to notice that the NGO's research practices were being changed in ways she found troubling. Its unique focus on people's experiences of participation, inclusion, and quality of life began to take a backseat to other interests. Sonya observed how the NGO's "rights" language gradually reformed over time and was incorporated alongside the growth and growing pressures and expectations placed on the organization.

This chapter relies on data (experiential and textual) from the lead author's work with the Right to Livelihood's Canadian-funded "Indicators Study," the report from that study, and Right to Livelihood's annual report data. Here we investigate how the insertion of dominant understandings of "the right to mental health and development" into organizational work processes was instrumental in that NGO's subtle and not so subtle shift to place "medical treatment" at the forefront of its model. The focus of our analysis is knowledge-making within Right to Livelihood, one of a very few organizations explicitly advocating for the rights of people in low-income countries experiencing "mental health problems." This approach is based on the Right to Livelihood's philosophy of building inclusive communities, involving so-called "mentally ill people" and their family and professional "caregivers" in the research process (NGO 2004).

Right to Livelihood's evolving research program, specifically the "Indicators Study," entered into what Smith (2006) called an intertextual circle of texts *informing* the Indicators Study. Description, field observations, and research reports all provided data for analysis. In our analysis we show how development practices (e.g., the exploration of indicators for measurement) and the dominant movement for global mental health (mGMH)— and goals of a rapid "scaling up" of mental illness diagnosis, treatment, and research—began to enter the way workers at the NGO understood and performed their work.

The Study's Practical and Contextual Background

This analysis does not take a position on the value, or lack of it, of the dominant health and development discourses. Rather, it highlights the *dominance* of particular concepts and activities and the subordination of others, as knowledge is being coordinated to meet goals for the "right to mental health and development." These are the diverse and distressing places on which those of us working in the current world of so-called global mental health practice must stand. We begin to explore the struggles from the starting place of the practical landscape of the NGO and conceptual landscape of the mGMH.

The Practical Landscape of Right to Livelihood's Participatory Research and Knowledge-Making

The lead author (Sonya) first met with the NGO in 2002 while teaching rural nurse practitioners in Northern Ghana. At that time, the NGO's Executive Director (ED), Ghana Programme Manager, and a field researcher, Amma, were conducting initial field consultations to determine whether and how the NGO might establish a program in Ghana. The founding organizational office is in the United Kingdom (UK) where the majority of program funding was obtained. Now, more than fifteen years since the NGO's origins, Right to Livelihood has offices that employ local managers and staff in several countries throughout the world, as well as separate Programme Management and Research offices at centralized locations. Right to Livelihood conducts "needs analyses" and field consultations with people deemed "mentally ill" as well as participating groups before establishing country programs in partnership with local stakeholders. As an organization, it is engaged in the complex relations of consulting with patients, families, caregivers,[4] and other community and government organizations, while also receiving funds and reporting back to external funding agencies.

The NGO's original participatory research approach includes a community consultation that involves psychiatrized people and caregivers in the research, analysis, and plans for utilizing the knowledge generated. The start of a consultation includes a community focus group (with people deemed "mentally ill," families, business owners, healthcare workers, and other stakeholders all participating). That consultation moves to smaller subgroups (e.g., groups of family or professional caregivers; distinct groups of men, women, children, and so on) who are all consulted about their unique concerns. Using a lifestory research approach, individuals and families are then interviewed and visited for more in-depth data collection.

Taken together, the consultation processes, lifestories, and all the consultation findings are analyzed in a participatory research process. Sometimes the very commonplace, or perhaps extreme, examples from the group consultations or the interviews will warrant greater exploration; thus, the process is iterative and unfolding. Regardless of the stories gathered, the work of the researchers in facilitating the consultations, lifestories, and participatory process is complex. Right to Livelihood's researchers have various kinds of investigative expertise; however, researchers like Amma all build relationships and trust in order to gather stories in the context of the unique individuals and communities.

One particular lifestory documented by Amma illustrates the research skills of group facilitation, participation, and observation involved—all necessary in the NGO's model. In this excerpt from lifestory records, she describes some of the context of the consultation and her focus on a particular family:

> It is a cold morning in [a northern Ghanaian primary school] and a group of over eighty people has congregated and settled in for the first participatory data analysis workshop, four months from the commencement of the [Right to Livelihood] programme in their district. We start to brainstorm the concepts of "data" and "data analysis." It is one of those moments when everybody just [sits] silently thinking about what these concepts could mean. This silence is however broken as [Mary Afua] and her mother walk into the room. The sound of shackles draws attention to Mary Afua's legs. Mary Afua is probably in her mid twenties and stands 5' 5" tall with a graceful stature. On this particular day, Mary Afua dons a dress, around which she wraps two colourful pieces of [cloth]. My attention again drifts to Mary Afua's aging mother whose face portrays years of worry. ... But again, as I look at the two, I marvel at how the pieces have been picked up after access to reliable treatment and a rejuvenated livelihood ... it is time to continue with the process of the day, so I refocus my thoughts on the proceedings of the workshop, but I am determined that we must listen to Mary Afua and her mother. (NGO Lifestory Records 2002, see Endnote 2)

Right to Livelihood incorporates these stories and the overall results of consultation into strategies to advocate for resources—including medical treatment—and services, to raise funds, and to illustrate public awareness and community education. Lifestory details of experiences labeled by the system as "mental illness" provide powerful messages and context. They give those previously stigmatized and marginalized a presence, however compromised, in circumstances in which they may otherwise have been misrepresented, or more misrepresented, or invisible. These stories are illustrative of the everyday language and struggles that are poorly captured by the official language of rights and other indicators. These stories also illustrate the tensions Right to Livelihood researchers must negotiate: creating awareness, raising funds, and listening to people.

Interviews with participants were transcribed and shared with everyone involved in the participatory process. The findings and thematic analysis of such participatory research played a pivotal role in the NGO's practice of building a case for fundraising, services development, and inclusion of participants into local vocational and health programs. For instance, Kofi's accounts (excerpted in what follows) of the impact of what he sees as his illness on his ability to work all factored into the later participatory analysis and testimonial documents for the NGO:

My sickness[5] affected many people. I was out of work because I thought it wise to get treatment before going back to work. This seriously affected our family income since it has not been easy to get an honest person to operate the tractor while I sought treatment. Farmers and traders who depended on my services had to turn to other sources amidst difficulties for tractor services. No man deserves this. Supposing you are with friends ... and this happens, you wake up stunned and confused. It disgraces and humiliates you. If you don't have a strong heart you may contemplate harming yourself, for example, attempting to commit suicide. (NGO Lifestory Records 2002, see Endnote 2)

Mary Afua and Kofi are both people with self-identified "mental health" problems who voluntarily participated in the Right to Livelihood's consultation process and lifestory research in order to have a voice in their communities; to raise their questions, concerns, and dilemmas; and to draw their own analyses on these matters in order to advocate for inclusion, support, and services. The NGO's approach captured our attention. We had been critically examining the role of research for mental health advocacy (Jakubec and Rankin 2014) and were following the critical discussions in the field that have been gaining momentum (Burstow et al. 2014; Ecks 2013; Mills 2014; Summerfield 2012). Despite our skepticism about the mGMH, the NGO's fundamentally inclusive and consultative process struck us as a unique contribution—one that offered a stark contrast to what we had observed, read, and written about in the critique.

Conceptual Landscape of the mGMH

To understand the disjuncture experienced by the lead author, and others in the field, one must understand the trends in psychiatry and a socially organized mGMH (Patel et al. 2008). The interests of mental health and development have evolved within a groundswell of discussion of global reforms for "mental health" infrastructure such as care frameworks (Thornicroft and Tansella 2013), treatment packages (Patel and Thornicroft 2009), skill packages with implementation rules (Swartz et al. 2014), and the use of performance measures (Marais et al. 2011). Perhaps the most important aspect of contemporary global mental health (GMH) discourse, and the focus of this institutional ethnography (IE) study, is the mGMH's interest in how human rights are central to knowing "mental health," and how human rights might count as evidence for decisions about resourcing (World Bank 2004, 2008).

GMH is currently used in conversations as a conceptual way of understanding "mental health" within processes for world health and development. The mGMH is tied into practices of the globalization of psychiatry (Fernando 2012) with what critical psychologists view as the imposition of Western understandings of individuation and personhood, biological explanations, and pharmacological interventions (Nelson and Prilleltensky 2002). The mGMH is also influenced by other practices of transcultural psychiatry (Prince 1991) and anthropologic approaches that seek cultural explanations and comparisons in place of universal constructs of illness.

The 1980s constituted an important milestone in the trajectory of the scale up of the mGMH (Shorter 1997); in particular, the publication of the revised version of the *Diagnostic and Statistical Manual of Mental Disorders* (DSM-III). The leading psychiatrists at the time hailed it as a revolutionary technology that would lead to "a victory for science" (Klerman et al. 1984, p. 539) and a reorganization and modernization of psychiatric diagnosis. Biomedicine and the pharmaceutical industry promoted the classification systems and played a pivotal role in mental health and development during these reforms (Kirk and Kutchins 1992).

According to Angell (2005), by 1980, the pharmaceutical industry was positioned to take off as the multinational and multimillion-dollar business it has now become. The pharmaceutical industry used DSM-III's "scientized" psychiatric message (American Psychiatric Association 1980) to promote drug research and medical interventions that remade psychiatric training and mental health practice (Moynihan et al. 2002). The new biomedical and psychiatric epidemiological discourse (Susser and Patel 2014) was widely adopted and had a globalizing influence (Jakubec and Campbell 2003).

The biomedical emphasis on "mental health" has had an important impact on how "global mental health" is being addressed. The mGMH's premise is that what are called, for example, depression and schizophrenia, are biological disorders no different from HIV-AIDS or epilepsy, and that people living in poor countries have just as much right to access effective drug treatments for mental disorders as people in "developed" countries (Patel et al. 2006). Despite the arguments of some experts claiming that drug treatments for psychiatric conditions are nowhere near as effective as believed (Summerfield 2008) and are even harmful (Kirsch 2009), those in the movement have relied on the appeal of equitable access to treatment to create the focus of the goals of the mGMH (Patel and Saxena 2014). What we see here is a conflation of human rights discourse and biological psychiatry discourse.

HUMAN RIGHTS AND COORDINATING EQUITABLE ACCESS TO TREATMENT

The emphasis on conventions and declarations for human rights (United Nations General Assembly 2007) by mGMH advocates is a more recent insertion into the agenda and rhetoric surrounding "mental health." With this emphasis on international conventions, the mGMH mirrors the seemingly successful movements for disability inclusion and HIV-AIDS treatment (Gable 2007). The successes of the HIV-AIDS human rights movement in attracting significant funding is seen as a perfect exemplar for people interested in advancing the mGMH (Ecks 2013).

Managing the Burden of "Mental Illness"

The economic "burden" of problems seen as mental illness is well documented in the literature (Whiteford et al. 2013), and the human rights imperative establishes a powerful argument for improved access to treatment (Wolff 2012). It is within these understandings that experts in the field saw financial resources as crucial to scaling up mental health services globally (Chisholm et al. 2007). According to Mills (2014), "[t]he discourse of burden is used here by the WHO and the mGMH to convey to governments (worldwide but particularly in LAMICs [low- and middle-income countries]) the need to increase spending and allocation of resources on mental health" (p. 29).

To understand the approach to managing the burden of disease through expanded access to treatment and the scaling up of the mGMH, it is crucial to grasp the "dollars, DALYs and decisions" (Chisholm et al. 2006, p. 7). This theoretical framework arose in the early 1990s as part of expanding "development" strategies and technologies for tracking the "global burden of diseases" (Desjarlais et al. 1996, p. 65). Disability-adjusted life years (DALYs) were pioneered by World Bank economists as an epidemiological tool that provided a way to measure years of lost productivity because of disease. Capacity to measure DALYs declared so-called "mental health problems" as a significant feature of global morbidity. The underlying belief of the mGMH within the burden of disease and disability conceptualizations is that "mental illness" is detrimental to development. This shift in focus resulted in the drive to calculate how much mental illness costs the national and international economy, and how much money could be saved by investing in effective drugs and competent personnel (Chisholm et al. 2006).

It is from this biomedical, psychopharmacological, and economic theoretical base that GMH is being scaled up (Eaton and Patel 2009). Current approaches to meeting the needs of people labeled "mentally ill" are framed by the availability of treatments, and how much an individual patient can afford to pay out of pocket for medications (Ecks and Basu 2009). Once accessed, "best treatment" is determined within standardized evidence-informed pathways and decision-making tools (Belkin et al. 2011). Under the mGMH rapid diagnoses and treatment are considered the highest standard (Patel et al. 2007). "Treatment" standards are derived from research conducted predominantly by the pharmaceutical industry, and in poor countries these choice treatments are listed in the WHO's 2009 report, *Pharmacological Treatment for Mental Disorders in Primary Health Care*. These grew from *The World Health Report 2001*, which emphasized: "Essential psychotropic drugs should be provided and made constantly available at all levels of health care. These medicines should be included in every country's essential drug list" (p. xi).

At all junctures, dominant ways of thinking about the right to mental health have become front and center. Several key areas of research have been identified "to inform the development of targeted and effective interventions in mental health care in Ghana" (Read and Doku 2012, p. 29), including aggressive poverty reduction and development approaches (Lund et al. 2011).

Efforts to finance strategic packages of "treatment" (Patel et al. 2007) have resulted in tightly planned training and service delivery options known as "pyramids of care" (Belkin et al. 2011, p. 1497) and rule-based implementation strategies. Such strategies dominate the direction that most GMH projects now take (Mills 2014). Broadly, leaders in the mGMH envision the achievement of scaled-up services through improved access to treatment with the expansion of trained community health workers (Thornicroft et al. 2012), and also through the improved research and administrative capacity (Marais et al. 2011) of community projects.

Current GMH theorizing and models of capacity-building all but ignore the fact that there already *is* a knowledge base (Ecks 2013). Outside of dominant GMH publications there is additional literature that articulates other perspectives of "mental health" rights, including antipsychiatry (Szasz 2010), "mad" studies (LeFrançois et al. 2013), and other critiques (Mills 2014; Summerfield 2008). Nonetheless, GMH, with its biomedical basis and emphasis on expanding access to rapid diagnosis and treatment internationally, has emerged as a dominant perspective in mental health and development activities.

Moving from Participatory Research to "Evidence" for the mGMH and Development

Within these practical and conceptual landscapes, the NGO leaders got the message that they would need to gather and analyze data in a different way, beyond the participatory research process they initially found successful, in order to expand their reach into other regions where people labeled "mentally ill" were suffering from stigma, being shunned, and experiencing a lack of services. As one of few international organizations advocating for mental health services, early in its inception leaders within mGMH held the Right to Livelihood up as a model program. The NGO's ED was invited to present and speak about the model at various international events and to contribute to other strategies and discussions. With this exposure came a pressure to more clearly identify and communicate what Right to Livelihood was accomplishing in the field.

Although none of the NGO's prior research practices included impact measures or calculative data, Right to Livelihood's leaders saw that they would need to expand the scope of their work to include a way of speaking about and measuring change in order to represent their model. More "rigorous research" with more refined areas of analysis would fit the NGO's desire for credibility and its Strategic Plan of 2003–2008 to expand the model (NGO Strategic Plan 2003, see Endnote 2).

This plan was a broad agenda to establish a more formal research department focused on specific goals related to research. The Strategic Plan included a Research Directorate based in South India where Right to Livelihood programs had been in operation the longest and where the largest database of process documents and community-based organization partners had been amassed. An expanded NGO Management Unit was established to support the coordinated efforts of internal data collection that could feed into more formal evidence and communication. The goals of widening the scope of the NGO's work in this way were the following:

[To] explore *in a collaborative programme of research* [emphasis added] the social, political and material contexts of mental health work in [the NGO's] programme countries. In each country setting the research will consider the contexts in light of relationships of policy, programmes and people's expressed needs. (NGO Strategic Plan 2003, p. 14; see Endnote 2)

"Scaling up" was part of Right to Livelihood's Strategic Plan that was vested in confronting the political roots of inequality that result in marginalization, exclusion, and control of people labeled mentally ill. To do this work more effectively, the Right to Livelihood leadership surmised that they needed to become more adept at producing evidence and influencing policy. Right to Livelihood's initial change indicators approach was developed from such evaluation and program development approaches as Weiss's theory of change (1995), which focused on identifying change indicators, including logical frameworks and logic models (Connell and Kubisch 1998).

Adopting this turn toward more "rigorous research," the NGO elaborated in its Strategic Plan (Right to Livelihood 2003, see Endnote 2) that they would explore indicators of change, conducting this work collaboratively and across programs internationally. Part of the NGO's Strategic Plan was to undertake an exploratory "change indicators" research project with Canadian and other partners. The Research Director, Rani, put it this way: "We can only work hard to make ourselves known, *producing evidence and presenting it in a way that can be heard* [emphasis added], that is what we are learning about policy making" (NGO Field Notes, Policy-Making Workshop Discussion 2005, see Endnote 2).

Producing evidence of sufficient rigor that would enable the NGO to credibly participate in discussions with policymakers and academics involved in the mGMH was a goal of the Right to Livelihood's Research Directorate (NGO Field Notes 2005, see Endnote 2). Thus, the NGO approached the growth of their Research Directorate and Management Unit strategically and in response to the development and the mGMH trends.

Being able to describe and define change indicators (in particular aspects of "mental health" or influencers on "mental health") became fundamental to the organization's new strategic agenda. Understanding and tracking these indicators was seen as a way to measure the impacts of the organization, effectively secure funds, and report to international granting agencies. Understanding the impact of its work in a measurable way, being able to look at trends internationally across program sites, and to produce numerical evidence or indicators of change all became part of the NGO's strategic evolution and plans.

For the Right to Livelihood, identifying change indicators would enable the organization to gather "better data" on what could count as impacts of their model and to communicate their findings with clarity and rigor. The NGO reported that the Indicator Study's goals were to "provide a framework to analyze the *impact* [emphasis added] of programme activities on the ground and assess [the NGO's] global influence in the mental health field" (NGO Six-Monthly Review 2005, see Endnote 2).

KNOWING INDICATORS OF "MENTAL HEALTH" AND DEVELOPMENT

The first proposal for international funding with the NGO's new Research Directorate was a small study to explore change indicators and to describe changes in mental health impacted by Right to Livelihood's participatory community consultation model. A proposal to the Social Sciences and Humanities Research Council of Canada (SSHRC) for an institutional grant was successful and was referred to as the Change Indicators Project or "Indicators Study." What follows is a textual analysis (Smith 2006) of the published study report that shows the subtle orientation toward "treatment" that it emphasized. It also shows how "treatment," a construction influenced by the emerging mGMH, would begin to predominate what the organization was to measure.

The "Indicators Study"

The Indicators Study research team proposed to explore Right to Livelihood program change indicators by analyzing existing focus group data from the NGO's Indian and Ghanaian consultations. Lifestory interviews, patient file data, as well as "process documents" were all part of the collected data. The team used the organization's participatory research model and theory of change frameworks (Weiss 1995) to assist in identifying the indicators of change from the data. They were interested in developing a way to understand the key areas of "mental health" and related influences that were seen to change in those involved in Right to Livelihood activities.

The NGO's ED, Research Director, and the first author of this chapter poured over the data and stories individually, in discussions via teleconferences, and in a week-long face-to-face workshop in Canada. The Indicators Study research team used the services of a Canadian university student to organize the data into spreadsheets that were categorized and highlighted to determine the dominant areas of change in "mental health" and various influencers. Although the research tasks were technical, the chart and document data reviews were emotional exercises. Seeing in print the lists of quotes from participants and "caregivers," the environmental and contextual concerns, and the poverty experienced by those who had attended consultations was compelling. The data motivated the research team's desire to study, disseminate, and build this case for mental health action within the NGO's programs and beyond.

Distilling Complex Lifestories and Experiences into Areas of Change and Impact

Being able to describe and define indicators also produced a way for the NGO to look at the trends that emerged over the first few years of the organization's work. The research team was able to review these intense circumstances and realities across sites in South Asia and Africa and to explore what was found in order to advocate for "mental health" needs and rights, as reflected in the data. The change indicators the research team identified were then crafted in an effort to capture the issues that arose in the data. Generating the indicators from numerous lifestories and organizational process documents gathered from consultations in India and Ghana was complex. As an example of the complexity, one of Amma's accounts we reviewed from a Ghana program lifestory was of a man, Kofi, who, estranged from his family, was living with 21 people in a guest house with no electricity or water. This piece of data graphically revealed the multiple challenges experienced in such a context:

> Because of the illness I stopped farming and did not have a source of income anymore. I also used to walk about aimlessly and got very tired. This [pointing to a broken door] is evidence that you can see for yourself. I knocked off the door and window under the influence of the illness. In a fit I also broke the glass compartment of my cupboard and it was on that day that my wife got scared and left with my three children to live with her parents. She is still married to me and hopes to return when my condition further improves. I hope for that. (NGO Lifestory—Kofi 2002, see Endnote 2)

In their analytic work to distil indicators of change from copious field data, the research team attempted to find a way to summarize the complex challenges of livelihood, household relations, and hope apparent in such lifestories. Even though they did not create categories by numerically coding key concepts, the indicators were a way to collapse what was wide-ranging. The following are the broad indicators of change the research team identified:

> 1. Impacts in the lives of poor mentally ill women, men, children and their families; 2. Change in policies, practices, ideas and beliefs; 3. Change in gender balance/equity; 4. Change in the involvement of mentally ill people and their family members in the project/program activity; and 5. The sustainability of change. (NGO Indicators Study Report 2003, see Endnote 2)

Although these five indicators of change attempted to hold the complexities and were not clearly measurable criteria, they became a standardized framework for the NGO's ongoing data collection and reporting across the international programs. There was nothing in the "Indicators Study" that specifically referenced biomedical treatment or access to treatment, although changes in policies, practices, ideas, and beliefs hinted at an interest in measuring health and social programs that included people labeled mentally ill and their families, or changes in beliefs about causation and treatment (e.g., that "mental problems" were caused by spiritual possession).

After completing the study, the research team reported on the identified indicators to the NGO fieldworkers in India and Ghana. This was done in order to "confirm" the identified categories and to discuss potential limitations or problems. Later in 2003 the indicators were field-tested by the organization. Inclusion of the indicators became a part of the NGO's routine project management system, working across country programs and general reporting activities. In addition, the indicators were used to provide speaking points and to create a shared language between emerging country program workers across the globe.

Adding Indicators into Right to Livelihood's Everyday Work

As a result of the "Indicators Study," changes were made between the NGO's Research Directorate and Management Unit so that overall reporting and "process documents" were formatted to bring in the internal indicators and to include current development and "mental health" language. The Indicators Study's texts contain clues that point back to the authorizing discourses and "boss texts." For example, impacts, equity, participant and stakeholder involvement, and sustainability were all listed as areas of reporting within the organization. Additionally, in the NGO's Annual Report (2003), the streamlining of its project management system highlights the alleged need for "stronger institutional measures" for the five indicators of change (p. 35, see Endnote 2). In this way the development of indicators were thought to fit within the organization's action research model and approach, while at the same time enabling more systematic collection of data, and more rigorous measures for internal management and external communication in line with the discourse of the GMH.

Internal reporting and field-testing (focus groups) with respect to the identified indicators occurred in 2003 with further review by the Research Directorate and another voluntary research associate. Partnering community-based organizations consistently reported that the "indicators" were relevant to the NGO's program work and promoted the interests and inclusion of the three key stakeholders (i.e., people deemed "mentally ill," families, and professional and community "caregivers"). The indicators "confirmed" that "treatment" played a crucial role in achieving the desired outcomes related to impacts on lives and in sustained changes in beliefs and policies, emphasizing that "the simplest way of effectively delivering improvement has been through regularly held field clinics where a professional provider of care commits to providing mental health services [treatment]" (NGO Annual Report 2003, p. 20; see Endnote 2).

Although the role of "treatment" was described in the original write-up of the "Indicators Study" as "a small part of the whole model for mental health and development" (NGO Indicators Study Report 2003, p. 10; see Endnote 2), it was an aspect of the model that supported the capacity to demonstrate that many of the indicators were being addressed. For instance, the numbers of people receiving treatment after a Right to Livelihood community consultation could stand as an example of the sustainability of change. Impacts of "treatment" (itself, note, a construction) with respect to what was deemed mental illness, correspondingly, were just one part, though an increasingly important part, of identifying the impact and sustainability of change. Nonetheless, in tandem with the discourses circulating in the mGMH and with the pressures to establish rigorous research, "psychiatric treatment" started to become more important to the overall NGO mandate. How did this happen?

New Evidence and Priorities for Scaling Up Right to Livelihood and the "mGMH"

Despite initial resistance, the adoption of the language of indicators—in particular, the emphasis on impact related to treatment and sustainability of treatment—was absorbed into the broad reporting at country program levels, as well as the local field levels, in all of Right to Livelihood's international programs. At the time of the NGO's annual reporting at the end of 2003, a shift toward the impact and achievement of sustainable treatment, and the links between treatment and employability and income, became visible in program reports. The following is from one such report emphasizing this:

> If the first theme of our consultations is access to health care, the second is renewed access to work and an income. One follows from the other. The stabilization that can be achieved through bringing people, often for the first time, to medical treatment, along with the support from both family and workers from our partner organizations, enables people once more to re-enter productive employment. (NGO Annual Report 2003, pp. 20–21; see Endnote 2)

Local community-based organizations and the NGO fieldworkers also began to discuss progress framed in terms of the indicators of treatment, productivity, and income; these were rapidly built into the participatory program review processes. When field-testing the "indicators," local community partner workers reported they could "clearly see change as more than a change in the illness condition alone" (NGO Indicators Study Report 2003, p. 10). In the project report, one local community-based organization leader was held up as an example of the usefulness of the indicators, pleased that he could now "quote *actual* examples that showed that stigma had been reduced" (NGO Indicators Study Report 2003, p. 9). This leader provided the NGO with other examples for the Indicators Study report, based on what he had heard on the ground from Ashok,[6] a man who was increasingly involved in community life, and for whom beliefs and quality of life were seen as indicators of change since Right to Livelihood's involvement in the community: "Earlier people in the village used to call Ashok 'mad.' They don't anymore ... Now he gets invited and attends marriages etc." (NGO Indicators Study Report, p. 10).

Change for another participant, Raj,[7] was expressed by a partner organization leader as follows:

> Earlier several people used to tell [local partner organization] staff, "Why are you dealing with this family. It's no use." Everyone had left them [abandoned the idea that anything could be done for them]. But now after seeing the changes they are all talking about it. Not only that, if there are jobs available [casual labour] they give first preference to Raj. (NGO Indicators Study Report, pp. 9–10)

The inclusion of people with "mental health problems" like Ashok and Raj into community life was a change that local community organizations and Right to Livelihood leaders—and, most fundamentally, families and those living with "mental health" problems themselves—observed.

These assessments are thoroughly aligned with the NGO's mandate. However, what was new was how the change indicators became increasingly linked closely with *treatment*, as evident in the NGO's 2003 Indicators Study report. Even though specifically naming social inclusion (e.g.., related to "livelihood" and "beliefs") in the report on the SSHRC Indicators Study, "the right to treatment" was highlighted as the starting place for these other indicators of change to take place. The NGO Indicators Study Report (2003), also emphasized the connection of "treatment" and "the right to treatment" to all manner of family relations, employment, and earning impacts:

> As for the families, they see treatment as a means to better cope with their burden of care—the burden magnified grossly by poverty. In an important addition, they see the possibility of the primary carer getting back to work, to being a wage earner thus *increasing the family's income as a consequence of treatment availability* [emphasis added]. (p. 11)

Throughout the Indicators Study report, the role of treatment was inserted as the "key" to unlocking change and success. Treatment, specifically, was identified as key to opening the door to social change for people and their problems:

> For mentally ill people, treatment appears to be the "key" [underline/emphasis present in the text] to their inclusion; the first and crucial step in their path from "exclusion to inclusion". They see treatment as making it possible for them to recover, earn and sustain their own livelihood and thereby having an increased role in the family and also realizing a larger social role through marriage (in several cases getting back with their spouses), family and community life. (NGO Indicators Study Report, p. 11)

This interpretation is closely aligned with the psychiatric mGMH discourse that dominates what can count as "evidence" of mental health needs, problems, and solutions (Ecks 2013; Mills 2014) that was circulating during the time the Indicators Study was being conducted.

Note how the sociocultural issues are attached to treatment transforming people's issues into by-products of *disease* rather than issues residing in the community, society, or political environments, what Jain and Jadhav (2009) referred to as "the pills that swallow [social] policy" (p. 60). The dominant mGMH and development discourses also are prominent in the summary of the Indicators Study, in which it is again emphasized:

> The first step in this process is exercising their [people with mental illness] right to treatment [underline/emphasis present in the text], realizing their health entitlements, which strengthens their ability to work and earn, thus capacitating them to realize their other rights and freedom to participate in family and community life. (NGO Indicators Study Report, p. 12)

The mGHM and development discourses concerned with the "right to mental health and development" are carried into the NGO's new change indicators.

In a paradoxical way this insertion of treatment introduced new individualized Western notions of rights as an entitlement (to biomedical treatment). These priorities overlook what Right to Livelihood had previously foregrounded—social, institutional, and political concerns that local community-based organizations and the NGO maintained were central to the mandates—that is, discrimination and exclusion and unequal access to self-help or state-provided assistance—discussed in the previous descriptive account of the NGO's work.

Despite the intentions in the Indicators Study to define change in an inclusive and consultative way, the indicators framework generated a *change measurement structure* with "treatment" identified as "key" and, as an extension, ameliorating the economic "burden of disease." To be clear, this "first step in the process" reflected in the NGO's Indicators Study did not arise from the data. Rather, it was selected from among the diverse interventions for "having a life" and reflects how the researchers' thinking was socially organized within the powerful ruling relations in the mGMH and development. It was firmly located in these discourses—first in terms of identifying disease in the individual, the "broken brain" (Andreasen 1984, p. 155), and then that it is a person's (individual) human right to access treatment and thus be equipped to work and contribute to productivity, decreasing the economic burden of disease.

The focus on people's abilities to earn and work reflects DALYs, "burden of disease," and the direction of those at the helm of the mGMH. The direction imparted by it is to aid in the economic development and productivity of "underproductive nations," now seen to be increasingly plagued by "mental illnesses" that rob individuals of the ability to participate in the globalized market economy. The mGMH discourse emphasizes that in resource-poor countries such as Ghana or India, "mental illnesses" should be addressed with efficient and "appropriate treatment" to support economic development.

This textual analysis of the Indicators Study illustrates how research work played a part in putting this mGMH frame into the Right to Livelihood's work processes. Attached to this frame were the Western economic language of

DALYs, "burden of disease," notions of productivity, and psychiatric diagnosis and treatment that are rolled into the common language of change indicators and sustained impact. Such practices subtly, and not so subtly, inserted different ways of knowing "mental health rights" that would coordinate with the NGO's growth, organizing the ways of recording its activities in new ways that more generally fit the scaling up of GMH.

Success in Widening the Canvas and Scaling Up GMH

The Indicators Study report was presented at an international health conference in October 2003. This presentation was for the Tenth Canadian Conference on International Health that had a theme called *The Right to Health: Influencing the Global Agenda—How Research, Advocacy and Action Can Shape Our Future* (Hatcher 2003). The report generated a great deal of interest. The research team presented it on the NGO's program with background, the impetus for the Indicators Study, and research methods, and its potential application to the change indicators. Conference participants appeared fascinated by the involvement of "mentally ill" people in knowledge-making and activism and on the emphasis on access to treatment. Unwittingly, nonetheless, the Indicators Study aligned with the medically trained audience and within the emerging mGMH context (Eaton et al. 2011) and human rights [as access to treatment] concepts built into the development discourse (Drew et al. 2011).

Opportunities for the NGO to continue its strategic work of expanding the research scope and reach were visible at the conference. The Indicators Study team met with an official Canadian international development research agency project manager. A newly developed funding unit at the agency aimed to support research that could strengthen equitable financing and delivery of health services, encourage citizen participation, and increase policy linkages. The NGO's early research efforts were a match with the funding unit's emerging emphasis on research into the right to health, user group participation in research processes, and the overall advocacy and policy objectives. A partnership with the Canadian agency was the next logical step forward for the Right to Livelihood to continue to advance its strategic research goals.

The NGO's work was seen by the Ottawa conference participants as a living, breathing example of the "right to health," the theme of the conference, and the application of approaches beyond the ideal and theoretical were unique examples at the time. The NGO's applications of inclusion and human rights into the model, and the distillation of this model into indicators that could be monitored and studied more rigorously, were tasks with which many other NGOs and government organizations and funders were grappling—that is, trying to understand both conceptually and practically. Demonstrating Right to Livelihood's program success in this way achieved the desired results and was met with a measure of success in terms of international reputation and spin-off possibilities. The Right to Livelihood's Strategic Plan for "scaling up" and disseminating findings were clearly in line with the budding trends and interests being expressed at this conference—the Indicators Study process had affirmed this aspect of the NGO's Strategic Plan.

Concluding Remarks

Completion of the initial Indicators Study and the presentation of this work at an international conference placed the Right to Livelihood on an international stage. Right to Livelihood began to organize more intensely around the goal of gathering good quality "evidence" in order to credibly and authoritatively communicate its success. Subtle changes were afoot. This led to an emphasis on the primacy of "treatment" and advancement of "the right to treatment" as crucial first steps for the NGO's participatory model. It also redirected the NGO's focus on livelihoods toward more specific "indicators," notions of the "economic burden" of care and disease, and "access to treatment."

In a follow-up to the Indicators Study, the organization also began to use logic model-driven evidence to reorganize its internal recordkeeping and project management work processes. It began to work newly configured "evidence" into what we also show as having an impact on the daily work of fieldworkers and local community-based organizations (Jakubec and Rankin 2014). It coordinated how they could continue to speak and write about their experiences with "mentally ill" people, "caregivers," and their circumstances in local communities. It shifted the organization away from its interest in "having a life" to being able to "earn a living" as a result of "getting treatment" (Jakubec 2015).

Textual analysis of the Indicators Study report provides a way to see how dominant development and mGMH frameworks started to be inserted into the NGO's way of understanding its own participatory model. Right to Livelihood's quest for evidence and the identification of indicators instituted a shift in priorities. This process moved Right to Livelihood in a research direction that established the groundwork for other projects. It drew the organization into the mGMH discourse in a way that paradoxically undermined its core mandate. We now have a grasp of how it is that this happened.

In conclusion, this chapter's authors should point out that besides what transpired with this particular NGO, the discourse of "indicators" and "right to treatment" play a more generalizable role in ruling health and development practice. The results of such a discourse are faced by people all over the world, those who wish to be understood, to understand what is happening to them outside of labels, and corresponding to prescribe treatment regimens for the mGMH.

Whereas diagnostic categories may support a certain grasp of a person's experience, these are always incomplete articulations; and they may operate so as to exclude people from the ranks of what is seen as normal in any society, as well as frequently culminating in actions that do people harm. In short, the power that these indicators give to the medical approach and psychiatrization is widespread; it is globalized in the mGMH; it itself creates distance and stigma—and it is unjustified.

NOTES

1. Throughout this chapter we are using this way ["mental health"] of referencing the emotional distress generally thought of as mental illness so as not to fall into what IE calls institutional capture; however, our referencing in this way should not be interpreted as taking a stand one way or the other on the validity of the concept of mental illness.
2. Pseudonyms and general terms are used for all proper and institutional names, both to respect the anonymity of those involved, and to acknowledge the generalizing features of the social organization of the discourse being explored. Whereas one specific account is examined here, the social organization extends far beyond the institutions and people described in this chapter.
3. All Right to Livelihood reports and documents have been omitted from the reference list to ensure participant anonymity. In some instances, a modified citation format has been used in order to include the title of the works.
4. Family and professional "caregivers" are also referred to as "carers" in the Right to Livelihood nomenclature.
5. In terms of official diagnoses, epilepsy is considered a neurological rather than psychiatric condition. In Ghana it is not commonly considered a "mental illness" per se; however, the practice is that patients with epilepsy typically are referred to psychiatric units.
6. Ashok was diagnosed as having schizophrenia for eight years before he began treatment.
7. Raj and his father both had "mental problems" that were untreated for more than two years, according to the local community-based organization staff; Raj had been severely ill. The family was considered destitute by the local community-based organization.

REFERENCES

American Psychiatric Association. (1980). Diagnostic and Statistical Manual of Mental Disorders. 3rd edition. Washington, DC: American Psychiatric Association.
Andreasen, N. C. (1984). The broken brain: The biological revolution in psychiatry. New York: Harper & Row.
Angell, M. (2005). The truth about the drug companies: How they deceive us and what to do about it. New York: Random House.
Belkin, G. S., Unützer, J., Kessler, R. C., Verdeli, H., Raviola, G. J., Sachs, K., et al. (2011). Scaling up for the "bottom billion": "5 x 5" implementation of community mental health care in low-income regions. Psychiatric Services, 62, 1494–1502. doi:10.1176/appi.ps.000012011.
Burstow, B., LeFrançois, B. A., & Diamond, S. (Eds.) (2014). Psychiatry disrupted: Theorizing resistance and crafting the (r)evolution. Montreal: McGill-Queen's University Press.
Chisholm, D., Saxena, S., and van Ommeren, M. (2006). Dollars, DALYs and decisions: Economic aspects of the mental health system. Retrieved from http://www.who.int/mental_health/evidence/dollars_dalys_and_decisions.pdf
Chisholm, D., Flisher, A. J., Lund, C., Patel, V., Saxena, S., Thornicroft, G., et al. (2007). Scale up services for mental disorders: A call for action. The Lancet, 370, 1241–1252. doi:10.1016/S0140-6736(07)61242-2.

Connell, J. P., & Kubisch, A. C. (1998). Applying a theory of change approach to the evaluation of comprehensive community initiatives: Progress, prospects, and problems. In K. Fulbright-Anderson, A. C. Kubisch, & J. P. Connell (Eds.), *New approaches to evaluating community initiatives, Volume 2: Theory, measurement, and analysis* (pp. 15–44). Washington, DC: The Aspen Institute.

Desjarlais, R., Eisenberg, L., Good, B., & Kleinman, A. (1996). *World mental health: Problems and priorities in low-income countries.* New York: Oxford University Press.

Drew, N., Funk, M., Tang, S., Lamichhane, J., Chávez, E., Katontoka, S., et al. (2011). Human rights violations of people with mental and psychosocial disabilities: An unresolved global crisis. *The Lancet, 378,* 1664–1675. doi:10.1016/S0140-6736(11)61458-X.

Eaton, J., & Patel, V. (2009). A movement for global mental health. *African Journal of Psychiatry, 12*(1), 1–3.

Eaton, J., McCay, L., & Semrau, M. (2011). Scale up of services for mental health in low-income and middle-income countries. *The Lancet, 378,* 1592–1603. doi:10.1016/S0140-6736(11)60891-X.

Ecks, S. (2013, August). *Panel summary—ethnographic perspectives on "global mental health."* Paper presented at the International Union of Anthropological and Ethnological Sciences – 17th Congress. Manchester, UK.

Ecks, S., & Basu, S. (2009). How wide is the 'treatment gap' for antidepressants in India?: Ethnographic insights in private industry marketing strategies. *Journal of Health Studies, 2,* 68–80 Retrieved from http://r4d.dfid.gov.uk/Output/190955/.

Fernando, G. A. (2012). The roads less traveled: Mapping some pathways on the global mental health research roadmap. *Transcultural Psychiatry, 49,* 396–417. doi:10.1177/1363461512447137.

Gable, L. (2007). The proliferation of human rights in global health governance. *The Journal of Law, Medicine & Ethics, 35,* 534–544. doi:10.1111/j.1748-720X.2007.00178.x.

Hatcher, R. J. (Chair). (2003, October). *Tenth Canadian conference on international health,* Canadian Society for International Health, Ottawa.

Jain, S., & Jadhav, S. (2009). Pills that swallow policy: Clinical ethnography of a community mental health program in northern India. *Transcultural Psychiatry, 46,* 60–85. doi:10.1177/1363461509102287.

Jakubec, S. L. (2015). *Knowing the right to mental health: The social organization of research for global health governance.* Conference abstract for the 34th International Congress on Law and Mental Health, July 12–17, 2015, Vienna, Austria.

Jakubec, S. L., & Campbell, M. (2003). Mental health research and cultural dominance: An analysis of the social construction of knowledge for international development. *Canadian Journal of Nursing Research, 35*(2), 74–88.

Jakubec, S.L., & Rankin, J.M. (2014). Knowing the right to mental health: The social organization of research for global health governance. *Journal of Health Diplomacy, 1,* 2. Retrieved from: http://www.ghd-net.org/journal-health-diplomacy-volume-1-issue-2

Kirk, S. A., & Kutchins, H. (1992). *The selling of DSM: The rhetoric of science in psychiatry.* New York: Aldine de Gruyter.

Kirsch, I. (2009). *The emperor's new drugs: Exploding the antidepressant myth.* London: The Bodley Head.

Klerman, G., Vaillant, G., Spitzer, R., & Michels, R. (1984). A debate on DSM–III. *American Journal of Psychiatry, 141,* 539–553.

LeFrançois, B. A., Menzies, R., & Reaume, G. (Eds.) (2013). *Mad matters: A critical reader in Canadian mad studies.* Toronto: Canadian Scholars Press.

Lund, C., De Silva, M., Plagerson, S., Cooper, S., Chisholm, D., Das, J., et al. (2011). Poverty and mental disorders: Breaking the cycle in low-income and middle-income countries. *The Lancet, 378*, 1502–1514. doi:10.1016/S0140-6736(11)60754-X.

Marais, D., Sombié, I., Becerra-Posada, F., Montorzi, G., & de Haan, S. (2011). *Governance, priorities and policies in national research for health systems in West Africa.* Geneva: Council on Health Research for Development.

Mills, C. (2014). *Decolonizing global mental health: The psychiatrization of the majority world.* New York: Routledge.

Moynihan, R., Heath, I., & Henry, D. (2002). Selling sickness: The pharmaceutical industry and disease mongering. *BMJ, 324*, 886–891.

Nelson, G. B., & Prilleltensky, I. (2002). *Doing psychology critically: Making a difference in diverse settings.* New York: Palgrave Macmillan.

Patel, V., & Saxena, S. (2014). Transforming lives, enhancing communities—innovations in global mental health. *The New England Journal of Medicine, 370*, 498–501. doi:10.1056/NEJMp1315214.

Patel, V., & Thornicroft, G. (2009). Packages of care for mental, neurological, and substance use disorders in low- and middle-income countries: PLoS Medicine series. *PLoS Medicine, 6*(10), e1000160. doi:10.1371/journal.pmed.1000160.

Patel, V., Saraceno, B., & Kleinman, A. (2006). Beyond evidence: The moral case for international mental health. *American Journal of Psychiatry, 163*, 1312–1315. doi:10.1176/appi.ajp.163.8.1312.

Patel, V., Araya, R., Chatterjee, S., Chisholm, D., Cohen, A., De Silva, M., et al. (2007). Treatment and prevention of mental disorders in low-income and middle-income countries. *The Lancet, 370*, 991–1005. doi:10.1016/S0140-6736(07)61240-9.

Patel, V., Garrison, P., de Jesus, M. J., Minas, H., Prince, M., & Saxena, S. (2008). The Lancet's series on global mental health: 1 year on. *The Lancet, 372*, 1354–1357. doi:10.1016/S0140-6736(08)61556-1.

Prince, R. (1991). Review of *From categories to contexts: A decade of the 'new cross-cultural psychiatry* by R. Littlewood. *Transcultural Psychiatric Research Review, 28*(1), 41–54.

Read, U. M., & Doku, V. C. K. (2012). Mental health research in Ghana: A literature review. *Ghana Medical Journal, 46*(Suppl. 2), 29–38.

Shorter, E. (1997). *A history of psychiatry: From the era of the asylum to the age of Prozac.* New York: John Wiley & Sons.

Smith, D. E. (2006). *Institutional ethnography as practice.* Toronto: Rowman & Littlefield.

Summerfield, D. (2008). How scientifically valid is the knowledge base of global mental health? *BMJ, 336*, 992–994. doi:10.1136/bmj.39513.441030.AD.

Summerfield, D. (2012). Afterword: Against "global mental health". *Transcultural Psychiatry, 49*, 519–530. doi:10.1177/1363461512454701.

Susser, E., & Patel, V. (2014). Psychiatric epidemiology and global mental health: Joining forces. *International Journal of Epidemiology, 43*, 287–293.

Swartz, L., Kilian, S., Twesigye, J., Attah, D., & Chiliza, B. (2014). Language, culture, and task shifting—an emerging challenge for global mental health. *Global Health Action, 7.* doi:10.3402/gha.v7.23433.

Szasz, T. S. (2010). Psychiatry, anti-psychiatry, critical psychiatry: What do these terms mean? *Philosophy, Psychiatry, & Psychology, 17*, 229–232.

Thornicroft, G., & Tansella, M. (2013). The balanced care model for global mental health. *Psychological Medicine, 43*, 849–863. doi:10.1017/S0033291712001420.

Thornicroft, G., Cooper, S., Van Bortel, T., Kakuma, R., & Lund, C. (2012). Capacity building in global mental research. *Harvard Review of Psychiatry, 20*, 13–24. doi:10 .3109/10673229.2012.649117.

United Nations General Assembly. (2007, January 17). 4th Session, Implementation of general assembly resolution 60/251 of 15 March 2006 entitled "Human Rights Council": Report of the special rapporteur on the right of everyone to the enjoyment of the highest attainable standard of physical and mental health, Paul Hunt, A/ HRC/4/28 . Retrieved from http://daccess-dds-ny.un.org/doc/UNDOC/ GEN/G07/102/97/PDF/G0710297.pdf?OpenElement

Weiss, C. H. (1995). Nothing as practical as good theory: Exploring theory-based evaluation for comprehensive community initiatives for children and families. In J. Connell, A. C. Kubisch, L. B. Schorr, & C. H. Weiss (Eds.), *New approaches to evaluating community initiatives: Concepts, methods, and contexts* (pp. 65–92). Washington, DC: Aspen Institute.

Whiteford, H. A., Degenhardt, L., Rehm, J., Baxter, A. J., Ferrari, A. J., Erskine, H. E., et. al. (2013). Global burden of disease attributable to mental and substance use disorders: Findings from the global burden of disease study 2010. *The Lancet, 382*, 1575–1586. doi:10.1016/S0140-6736(13)61611-6.

Wolff, J. (2012). *The human right to health*. New York: Norton.

World Bank. (2004, August). *Mental health and the global development agenda: What role for the world bank*. Retrieved from http://siteresources.worldbank.org/ INTPH/Resources/376086-1256847692707/6526326-1287681563483/ RachelMentalHealth.pdf

World Bank. (2008). *Mental health patterns and consequences: Results from survey data in five developing countries* (Policy Research Working Paper No. WPS4495). Retrieved from doi:10.1596/1813-9450-4495

CHAPTER 7

Pathologizing Military Trauma: How Services Members, Veterans, and Those Who Care About Them Fall Prey to Institutional Capture and the DSM

On August 28, 2014, Master Corporal Denis Demers, a medical technician who had been with the Canadian Armed Forces (CAF) for 12 years and who had recently completed two tours in Afghanistan, barricaded himself inside his home and indicated that he was intending to take his own life. After receiving a call from concerned family members, military police and Ontario Provincial Police officers showed up at the house. An almost 40-hour-long standoff ensued and ended two days later when police took Demers into custody and proceeded to admit him to the psychiatric ward of a local hospital. Corporal Demers was released 24 hours later. On September 12, two weeks after the standoff, Demers killed himself, leaving behind a wife and four young sons. His body was found outside his home near Canadian Forces Base Petawawa in Ontario. Almost all media accounts of this story suggest Demers was experiencing posttraumatic stress disorder (PTSD).

Corporal Demers's story is similar to countless others across Canada and the United States; it also highlights three key disjunctures. The first is the fact that an increasing number of Canadian Armed Forces members are killing themselves. In fact, in September 2014, the government of Canada released

L. Spring (✉)
University of Toronto, Toronto, Canada
e-mail: lauren.spring@mail.utoronto.ca

© The Editor(s) (if applicable) and The Author(s) 2016   125
B. Burstow (ed.), _Psychiatry Interrogated_,
DOI 10.1007/978-3-319-41174-3_7

a troubling statistic: In the past decade, Canada lost more members of the CAF to suicide than it did on the battlefield in Afghanistan (Campion-Smith 2014a). A total of 138 Canadian soldiers were killed in combat between 2002 and 2014, whereas between 2004 and 2014, 160 committed suicide. The statistics are particularly striking when one considers that the numbers in question do not take into account suicides among veterans but only reflect regular forces' members and reservists. In the United States, the numbers are even more staggering. In 2014 alone, more than 434 service members killed themselves (Childress 2015). From 2001 to 2013, more than 2700 active-duty service members (discounting those from the National Guard and reserve troops) took their own lives (Dao and Lehren 2013).

The second disjuncture is that the powerful institutions that make up the relations of ruling (i.e., in this case the medical system, the media, and the military itself) continue to portray all CAF members and veterans who are having problems with living as "mentally ill." Because of this fact, record numbers of military men and women are being diagnosed with and "treated" for PTSD and other putative disorders found in the *Diagnostic and Statistical Manual of Mental Disorders* (DSM). In spite of much evidence to the contrary, the ruling groups continue to perpetuate the idea that it is a "mental illness" to be traumatized by war and military service, and that most suicides are the result of a "mental illness"—namely, PTSD.

This line of thinking has inspired countless educational and destigmatization campaigns run by PTSD-awareness organizations. Such campaigns suggest that *if only* more "help" would be made available, *if only* those with "mental illness" would not fear reaching out for "professional help," and/or *if only* governments would increase the military mental health budget, these tragedies could be prevented. Trauma from military service, however, is a great deal more complicated than the psychiatric regime of ruling and PTSD-awareness organizations make it out to be; most military men and women who kill themselves are compelled to do so not because they are "mentally ill" but because they are having difficulty connecting with family members and friends, finding steady employment, and transitioning out of a military culture into civilian life (Dao and Lehren 2013; Hale 2015; Monson et al. 2009; Nazarov et al. 2015).

This brings one to the third disjuncture: The "treatment" that service members and veterans receive for PTSD and other DSM disorders—that is, the "help" they are offered—commonly causes great, irreversible harm. As will be explained here, in many cases it is not the trauma at all but the effects of the "treatment" itself that drive people to take their own lives.

This chapter outlines the origins of PTSD as a "disorder"—one that, ironically, veterans themselves lobbied to have included in the DSM—and explores the ways its existence is regularly perpetuated through the ruling relations. It then traces how (and why) healthcare workers, soldiers, veterans, and those who care about their well-being, "activate" the language of the DSM as part of their everyday work—even though it does them a tremendous disservice.

GATHERING DATA

For this research, in addition to reading countless newspaper articles, government-issued documents, and psychiatric reports, I conducted three in-person interviews with "medical professionals" who specialize in working with the traumatized military population on a daily basis. One is a social worker, another a psychologist, and the third is a top military psychiatrist with the Canadian Armed Forces. I also conducted an online interview with an employee at the Royal Canadian Legion—an organization that assists veterans with a great many tasks, including making disability claims and seeking compensation from the government for their injuries.

This was augmented using a virtual strategy. I used as a primary source of data, posts and comments made by members of the public (e.g., a vast majority of veterans or family members of service members or veterans) on two popular military support group Facebook pages: Military Minds and Military with PTSD. I reviewed all posts made by site administrators, and all comments these posts produced between September 2010 and July 2015. Such posts are cited similar to other anonymous interviews with a reference to the cases available at https://www.facebook.com/MilitarywithPTSD/?fref=ts and https://www.facebook.com/MilitaryMindsInc/?fref=ts, respectively.

I should add here that while traditional institutional ethnography (IE) research primarily focuses on tracing *how* disjunctures occur (and the following pages strive to do exactly that), I also at times—because my data was rife with examples—suggest *why* this may be happening so that it is possible to better understand how and where changes could occur.

THE "BOSS TEXT" AND PTSD

Before tracing exactly how the language of the DSM is activated currently, it is important to understand how "PTSD" first came to be included in the DSM several decades ago. As a diagnostic category, posttraumatic stress disorder has existed only since 1980—the year it was first included in the DSM-III (Boone 2011; Cukor et al. 2009). Up until that point, military trauma was viewed in a variety of ways. During the First World War (WWI), for example, soldiers displaying strange and unusual behavior were considered "shell shocked," and it was believed their behavior was a result of "concussions caused by the new high explosives used in battle" (Boone 2011, p. 2).

A diagnostic shift took place in 1943 when the US government, realizing they had spent more than a billion dollars on caring for the psychiatric needs of WWI veterans, shifted the blame onto the victims and began to label their problems with living as "war neurosis"—a condition thought to be caused by "inherent weakness or defective parenting and (only) aggravated by armed conflict" (p. 2). The US government and military (then, no longer responsible for having caused the trauma) considered themselves off the hook in terms of follow-up treatment and therapy and were quick to discharge any soldier "displaying psychiatric distress of any kind" (Boone 2011, p. 2). As the Second World War (WWII) continued and as the United States found itself with an acute lack of manpower, the idea of "combat exhaustion" emerged. This implied that military trauma was in fact not a "deep-seated pathology" that required immediate discharge from the military but was merely circumstantial and could be treated with "rest, emotional support, and encouragement" over several weeks, after which soldiers could return rather quickly to battle (Boone 2011, p. 2).

The concept of "combat fatigue," however, had no real parallel in civilian psychiatry and was thus awkwardly incorporated into the category of "gross stress reaction" when the DSM was first published in 1952. In the second edition published 16 years later, though, the category of "gross stress reaction" was removed, thereby leaving psychiatrists without a clear model with which to better diagnose soldiers who had endured extreme stress; thus, many military personnel were left without the "professional" help they felt they needed (Boone 2011).

The inclusion of PTSD in the DSM-III published in 1980 was largely a result of lobbying efforts on the part of US Vietnam veterans who felt that the American Psychiatric Association (APA) needed to create a diagnosis so that their (veterans') "long-term psychological damages" could be recognized (Burstow 2005, p. 430). Such a recognition, it was thought, would also "pave the way for therapeutic services" veterans felt they needed (p. 430); this was initially seen as a positive step in terms of the government being forced to acknowledge the role that it had played in contributing to the trauma (as it then was up to it to compensate veterans and help pay for "treatment").

Since the 1980s and the publication of the DSM-IV in 1994 and DSM-5 in 2013, the diagnostic criteria related to PTSD have undergone several significant transitions. As a result of these shifts in language and criteria, a record number of people (e.g., not only soldiers and veterans but also sexual assault victims and those who have survived natural disasters or vehicle accidents) receive a diagnosis of PTSD each year.

Government statistics indicate that between 2002 and 2014 "depression" was the diagnosis most commonly ascribed to Canadian military personnel (Pearson et al. 2014). An article entitled "Mental Health of the Canadian Armed Forces" describes results from the 2013 Canadian Forces Mental Health Survey (CFMHS) that indicate that 8 % of regular CAF members reported "symptoms" of depression that year compared to 5.3 % who reported "symptoms" of PTSD. More recent statistics, however, show that PTSD is fast becoming the most common diagnosis among CAF members and veterans; in fact 25 % of those deployed to "combat heavy zones" in Afghanistan between 2001 and 2008 received a diagnosis of PTSD within four years of returning home (Nazarov et al. 2015, p. 5).

Charles Hoge, one of the few military doctors who seems capable of adopting something close to the achieved standpoint of military men and women—he is highly critical of psychiatry in general and PTSD in particular—has also identified that "PTSD has gained a much higher level of importance during the wars in Iraq and Afghanistan than in any prior conflict" (Nazarov et al. 2015, p. 1). In a conversation with one interviewee, I inquired about why, in spite of the fact that rates of depression in military circles have been much higher than those of posttraumatic stress disorder over the past decade, PTSD is the disorder grabbing public attention.

I also asked why the interviewee thought rates of PTSD diagnoses are on the rise. He suggested that it likely comes down to the question of attribution, as follows:

> PTSD ... can very easily be politicized. Because this is what you've done to people. A government has sent people to war and look what's happened, they come back broken. ... Schizophrenia just sort of happens, depression often too but with PTSD—there is this attribution to this traumatic event. On the surface there's a really clear cause-and-effect kind of idea. So you sent Johnny to war, Johnny got blown up, Johnny is now having nightmares and flashbacks, therefore you sending him caused this. Therefore you have to solve this. It's your problem. (Personal communication, May 18, 2015)

In large part it seems that it is this sense of attribution that continues to drive the activation of language from the DSM. On some level this seems like a good thing, but not when it is misunderstanding and harm that is engendered.

That noted, the coming sections will illustrate how the military, media, and psychiatric system activate this "boss text" in a variety of ways that profoundly influence the ways service members, veterans, and those who care about them frame their experiences and behaviors. Even though public discussions about the mental health of military and veteran populations may seem positive at first blush, pathologizing complex and nuanced feelings and experiences as "symptoms" of PTSD is causing devastating, long-lasting harm to the very people it purports to help.

THE CONSTRUCTION OF "PTSD-RELATED SUICIDES"

As Figure 7.1 illustrates, the idea of PTSD—stemming from the DSM—is activated primarily by three different groups within the ruling relations: the media, the military, and psychiatry. As the figure also shows, texts produced by all three are somewhat intertwined and influence one another in a circular fashion. For example, newspaper articles and television programs that sensationalize the increase in military suicides influence the military's personnel to make decisions to produce new texts that relate to internal "PTSD education" programs, public awareness, and de-stigmatization campaigns. Such texts in turn encourage more members and veterans of the CAF to seek psychiatric "help" that in turn increases the number of military PTSD diagnoses nationwide over time; this is a phenomenon on which the media will surely report, sparking another response from the military—and the cycle continues.

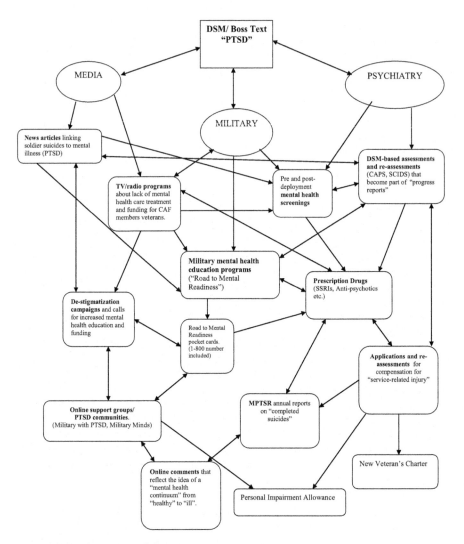

Figure 7.1 Activation of the DSM

One would be hard-pressed these days to find a newspaper article on the subject of military suicides that does not also address "rising rates of PTSD" (Dreazan 2014). For example, a 2014 article in the *Globe and Mail* opens by citing the statistic that "the rate of post-traumatic stress disorder among members of the Canadian Forces has nearly doubled since 2002," and it goes on to say that "a rash of returning soldiers' suicides raise[s] questions about the Canadian military's ability to cope with the psychological fallout of the Afghanistan mission" (Grant 2014). In another example, Mackenzie (2014) in an article, also from the *Globe and Mail*, states:

The greatest hurdle to preventing suicide is getting the individual[s] to recognize that they have a mental-health problem … [For] the vast majority of soldiers committing suicide, … the mental illness went unidentified by fellow soldiers, leadership and medical professionals and the opportunity for treatment was missed. (p. XX)

This linking of military suicide to "mental illness" was also very apparent in all media accounts about Cpl. Denis Demers's death—the story referenced at the start of this chapter. For example, a CTV news report followed up its account of the facts of Demers's situation with the comment: "family and friends believe he was suffering from PTSD" and then proceeded to conduct an interview with Joseph Jorgensen, the executive director of Military Minds Inc. The newscaster introduced Jorgensen by saying: Military Minds believes that Denis Demers "was ill and did not get the help he needed." As the interview progresses, the reporter asks him: "Do they believe he (Demers) was suffering from Post-Traumatic Stress Disorder and that's what led to his suicide?" Jorgensen then responds by saying, "I can't comment on that, but I believe … it's apparent" ("Canadian Soldier…," Video 2014).

Such comments are especially troubling considering the fact that during his lifetime (and 12 years in the CAF), whether or not Demers received a diagnosis of PTSD was not public knowledge. This fact, however, did not stop the media from pathologizing his actions posthumously. Suggesting it must have been Demers's (officially nonexistent) PTSD that compelled him to kill himself is not only misguided but also ignores the myriad of personal and professional reasons that usually drive someone to take his own life—reasons that have nothing at all to do with "mental illness." For example, the 2015 Medical Professional Technical Review (MPTSR) report itself—a report in which all suicides by CAF members are reviewed for a complete calendar year—indicates that 75 % of those who killed themselves during 2013 reported relationship failure, 42 % were struggling with financial problems, and 50 % had career difficulties (Herber and Roux 2015).

Additionally, the findings of a report published in *JAMA Psychiatry* suggest that suicide might have much more to do with feelings of dishonor and lack of heroism than the nightmares and flashbacks considered "symptoms" of PTSD in the DSM (Kime 2015a; Philipps 2015). In fact, many details of this report run contrary to the PTSD discourse. For example, it cites that deployment over long periods of time may actually *lower* members' suicide risk. In this regard, the study found that the suicide rate for troops who left the military before completing a four-year enlistment was nearly twice that of troops who stayed in longer. The rate for troops who were involuntarily discharged under less-than-honorable conditions for disciplinary infractions was nearly three times higher (Philipps 2015).

In spite of this evidence, countless newspaper articles and radio and television interviews continue to perpetuate the myth that PTSD exists, is a "mental illness," and is the cause of most military suicides. Such reports are not innocuous. There is an overarching storyline that pervades the media that *if only* more individuals were properly diagnosed and sought professional help, *if only* the media and the public could work together to "de-stigmatize" PTSD and other "mental illnesses," these suicides could be prevented. To this end, newspaper articles often provide links to "helplines" and referral services for readers who think they themselves or a loved one in the military may be suicidal or in need of help (Brewster 2013; Tucker 2014).

"Mental health" has become a priority for the military over the past decade, and the Department of National Defence (DND) has been working closely with psychiatrists to develop specialized programs and assessments for the armed forces. Members of the Canadian Armed Forces are familiarized with the idea of PTSD early on in their training because all CAF personnel undergo regular pre- and post-deployment "mental health screenings." For more comprehensive information on which CAF members are screened and when, please refer to the DND's "PTSD backgrounder" ("Post-traumatic Stress Disorder," n.d.). There also are efforts underway to screen (and not accept for service) those who might be susceptible to PTSD or suicide before they join the military (Nazarov et al. 2015).

Once in the army, service members are constantly reminded that mental illnesses are "real" and instructed to look out for "symptoms" in themselves and their buddies. Since 2009, when the Canadian government first implemented the "Road to Mental Readiness" (R2MR) program, more than 56,000 CAF members "have received some sort of mental health training and education" ("Suicide...," n.d.). Service members receive R2MR education during basic training, during all leadership training, and pre- and post-deployment.

As shown earlier in Figure 7.1, CAF members also are given R2MR pocket cards, presumably so that they can keep them on their person. The card itself outlines a "Mental Health Continuum" that ranges from "healthy" to "ill" and describes symptoms and behavior for each stage of the continuum, supposedly so that soldiers can self-assess when on the battlefield or after returning home. For example, if one "cannot fall/stay asleep" or is "absent from social events," these are symptoms that one is on the extreme "ill" end of the continuum and, as such, they are advised to "seek consultation" and a 1–800 number is supplied on the card.

Nearly all DND resources on the subject also clearly link suicides with mental illness—PTSD especially. For example, the Canadian Armed Forces Department of Defence official "Suicide Prevention" webpage states:

> Every suicide is a tragedy, including the loss of any of our soldiers. ... The CAF's extensive mental illness awareness and suicide prevention measures consist of clinical and non-clinical interventions by generalist and specialist clinicians, mental health education, and suicide awareness information. ... We each have a role to play in identifying and assisting those affected by mental illness. Once we are collectively educated and able to recognize the onset of mental illness, we can help

our friends, colleagues and family members by encouraging care. ... The CAF remains committed to reducing the barriers that may interfere with obtaining timely mental [health] care. Stigma is one of these barriers. Through dialogue, training and leadership, we can create a culture in which care seeking is encouraged and facilitated. ("Suicide...," n.d.)

Again, here we see the assertion that suicides by military personnel are caused by "mental illness" and the suggestion that if an individual having problems with living seeks "professional" care, and receives a diagnosis and follow-up treatment in a timely manner, one's suicide will likely be prevented. This ideology, popularized far and wide, ignores the fact that the "help" to which these documents refer actually does not seem to be helping those in distress much at all. In fact, according to the 2015 MPTSR report, of the 12 recorded suicides in 2013 for which reports were written up, 7 of these individuals *had* received a mental health diagnosis (i.e., PTSD, major depressive disorder, or anxiety disorder), and they *were* in the "system" and in the process of "receiving treatment" when they decided to take their own lives (Herber and Roux 2015).

It is important to remember here that the MPTSR report only looked at suicides of active-duty CAF members; this report is the most recent, and it documents 13 suicides in 2013. Thus, suicides committed by veterans—whose health concerns often fall through the cracks—are not counted here (Campion-Smith 2014b). This means that these active-duty individuals who killed themselves in 2013 would not have had to wait weeks for care or attention, nor would they have had to worry about the financial burden of paying for "treatment" (complaints we often hear of from veterans). No, these individuals would have had access to the "best possible system in Canada" in a very timely manner (personal communication, May 18, 2015).

The report also states that 50 % of those who killed themselves also had made previous suicide attempts of which their health teams were aware. One interviewee reaffirmed during our discussion that the federally overseen healthcare program to which CAF active-duty service members have access is the "gold standard" of healthcare in Canada:

We built our own health care system. ... We have our own electronic health record, we sort out our own pharmacy, our own drugs. We have our own leadership, our own policies ... the whole thing. So we built the mental health program that we felt we needed. ... What we have built is an outstanding system. ... We have built something that we consider the gold standard. (Personal communication, May 18, 2015)

If this perception is true, the question arises: Could some soldiers have killed themselves not *in spite of* the treatment they were receiving, but *because of* its effects? Should not the fact that more than half of the CAF members who killed themselves in 2013 were receiving "the best care this country has to offer" at the time of their suicides be an indication that the current system is not working?

As shown in Figure 7.1 earlier, it is significantly more difficult for veterans to find "help" when they need it than it is for active-duty service members. As mentioned, the CAF does not keep track of how many veterans kill themselves in the country each year. In the United States, however, Veteran's Affairs (VA) currently estimates that as many as 22 veterans commit suicide each day (Dao and Lehren 2013). Typically, if Canadian veterans are experiencing distress (e.g., nightmares, etc.), they will be referred to an Operational Stress Injury Clinic for assessment.

One interviewee told me that the most common assessments used for military patients at these clinics and elsewhere are the Structured Clinical Interview for DSM Disorders (SCIDS) and the Clinician Administered PTSD Scale (CAPS). Receiving a DSM diagnosis makes a veteran eligible to apply for financial compensation—either as a lump sum under the New Veterans Charter (NVC) or in the form of a Permanent Impairment Allowance. A representative from the Royal Canadian Legion pointed out that in order to receive a Permanent Impairment Allowance a veteran must be considered "severely disabled as a result of PTSD" (Personal communication, April 22, 2015). To qualify for this, veterans typically have to be reassessed by a psychiatrist on a semi-regular basis to confirm that they are still disabled by their PTSD and qualify to continue to receive benefits.

Even though it is, in these cases, understandable and financially advantageous for veterans and their doctors to activate the language of the DSM, such activations can have dire consequences. The next section of this chapter traces some of these consequences. Charles Hoge (2010) argues that while "PTSD has become part of the vocabulary of modern warriors" (and while the military, psychiatry, and the media view this as a positive step), we must be wary of the ways it is being "misused as a catchall term for *any* postwar behavioral problem" (p. 1). The more that military personnel, veterans, and those who care about them continue to fall prey to institutional capture and to uncritically embrace and activate the language of the DSM, the more bureaucratic and less nuanced and human "treatment" approaches will become.

ACHIEVED STANDPOINT AND WHY "NO ONE COMMITS SUICIDE"

In a compelling article entitled "No One Commits Suicide: Textual Analysis of Ideological Practices," Smith (1983) uses Virginia Woolf's suicide (and the media and other text-based accounts of it) to illustrate how regimes of ruling pathologize ordinary human behavior. Smith suggests that words like "suicide" are part of an "abstracted system of representing 'what happened/what is' in which the subject is canceled" (Smith 1983, p. 311). The expression "she killed herself," Smith argues, reflects the actuality of the experience itself, whereas saying "she committed suicide ... embeds the story in the relations of ruling" (p. 311).

One finds a similar abstracting of reality when reviewing official military documents, summaries, and recommendations on cases of CAF members who have killed themselves. There are several striking examples of this in the most recent MPTSR report set forth by the DND (Herber and Roux 2015). The report itself is strikingly impersonal; the document never once states that an individual "killed himself/herself" but rather classifies these deaths as "completed suicides." Similarly, while certain details of these deaths are examined and reported on (e.g., the "most common method of suicide" is "hanging"), the human factors—the complexities that lead individuals to kill themselves, and what differentiates one from another—are noticeably absent.

The report indicates that 6 out of 13 hung themselves, 3 used a firearm, 3 others died of asphyxiation (e.g., "carbon monoxide, drowning, or helium-induced"); for one the method was "unknown"—statements were written up for only 12 of the 13 deaths (Herber and Roux 2015, p 2). Similarly, though three regular forces women killed themselves in 2012, and one killed herself in 2013, the loss of their lives were not included in official government statistics because the numbers tended to be "too small" and thus were deemed statistically insignificant ("Suicide...," n.d.).

This chapter, in taking on the achieved standpoint of a soldier or veteran traumatized by military experience, attempts to humanize the statistics and to move away from what Smith (1983) refers to as the "ideological schema of mental illness" (p. 350) by bringing the individual and his or her work and actions in specific places and at specific times back to the center of the discussion. For this reason, I have opted to use the expression "killed herself/himself" instead of the more abstracted phrase "committed suicide" wherever possible.

Taking a standpoint that begins in the body, one that "works from the actualities of people's everyday lives and experience to discover the social as it extends beyond experience" (Smith 2005, p. 10), is particularly appropriate when working with military personnel. Soldiers' bodies have been through a great deal. Basic training alone requires that all members pass an intense initial physical fitness evaluation; often they must wake up at 5 a.m. each morning to participate in 90 minutes of weight lifting, running, forced marches, and/or other physical training. If deployed, soldiers may lose limbs from the force of explosions brought about by improvised explosive devices (IEDs) or rocket attacks. During a Canadian mission in Afghanistan, more than 6 % of the soldiers on the ground were reported to have suffered a traumatic brain injury (Sher 2011).

CAF veteran and artist Scott Waters, in a short illustrated memoir he calls the *Hero Book* (2006), vividly recalls (17 years after the event) a day at Battle School where he was made to bite into the neck of a live bird:

As my teenage teeth sank into the grouse's neck I was mostly surprised at how warm and soft it was. (Imagine biting into a heated, feathery Twinkie.) Perhaps the hollow bones helped. Though much has faded, I can close my eyes right now (right now) and feel the warmth, the fuzziness and the ease with which I performed my first kill for the infantry. (p. 35)

What relates to this, numerous military personnel I've met and interviewed over the years have a conspicuous way of standing at attention when greeting new people and of darting through traffic on foot to meet me across a busy street—an audacity that I've not witnessed among ordinary civilians.

Military training stays in the body. Trauma does too. For example, the Military with PTSD organization recently launched a campaign. (I used this Facebook group as a primary source of data for this research.) In the lead-up to the US 4th of July celebrations, they organized sending out more than 2500 lawn signs to veterans across the country. The signs read: "Combat veteran lives here, please be courteous with fireworks"; this was done because many veterans say that the sound of fireworks triggers intense flashbacks to the battlefield.

Most psychiatrists would interpret this reaction to fireworks as a "symptom" of PTSD; however, Hoge (2010) sees it differently and reminds veterans that the alleged "flashbacks" are simply a result of intense military training; he also observes that many things that medical professionals label "symptoms" are actually "combat survival skills" service men and women were trained to exhibit—"hyperarousal" is a prime example (p. 9). Such a state is necessary in battle, and it is only normal that such reactions should persist into civilian life. Which brings us to: What happens to veterans and service members so diagnosed?

Drugs' Effects, Frustrations, and Institutional Capture

During the interviews that I conducted for this chapter, it became strikingly clear that the vast majority of individuals who receive a PTSD diagnosis are given prescription drugs as a first course of "treatment." I will be focusing on the results of this in the coming pages. The concentration will be expressly on the "work" soldiers and veterans do on a daily basis, as reflected in their posts and comments on online support groups. For institutional ethnographers, "work," note, includes not only paid employment but also "anything and everything people do that is intended, involves time and effort, and is done in a particular time and place and under definite local conditions" (Smith 2006, p. 10).

As this section illustrates, the "work" being done by veterans and those purporting to advocate on their behalf often ends up activating the language of the DSM. This is so especially when it comes to discussions about prescription drugs; much of the work people do and advise others to do leads down a dangerous path that can adversely affect veterans' amorous and familial relationships, employment opportunities, and financial situations—the main factors that, according to the MPTSR report, compel people to kill themselves.

To begin with the interviews: Two interviewees who work closely with those diagnosed with PTSD noted that "almost all" of the military men and women they see are on one type of prescription drug or another. One interviewee responded that he did not think he had "ever seen a military guy or woman in the program who wasn't on some sort of medication" (Personal communication, October 30, 2014). The other interviewee justified it thus:

> If a patient's anxiety is so high that they can't really engage with some of the behavioral stuff, if they are so overwhelmed by an emotional experience that they can't even organize themselves to do any of the grounding or tolerate the imaginable exposures because the contact with that memory is just so overwhelming, there is a role for medications for sure. So I'm, I ... I look at them [drugs] not as a solution but as a way to sort of facilitate the engagement of the psychological process." (Personal communication, January 28, 2015)

All interviewees also pointed out to me that currently there are not actually any specialized drugs to treat PTSD. Many of the drugs being used today are selective serotonin reuptake inhibitors (SSRIs), which are commonly prescribed for depression and anxiety disorders. According to the US Department of Veteran's Affairs, SSRIs are "the only medications approved by the Food and Drug Administration for PTSD" ("Professional Treatment Overview," n.d.). Although some soldiers claim that these drugs "can take the edge off debilitating symptoms" (Hoge 2010, p. 199), they also bring with them a whole host of negative effects including increased anxiety, gastrointestinal problems, and sexual dysfunctions as well as "... irritability, paranoia, delusions, confusion, impulsivity..." (Burstow 2015, p. 336).

In many cases men on various types of SSRIs become impotent or have great difficulty reaching orgasm—that can be frustrating for them and their sexual partners and may contribute to relationship troubles (again, the leading cause of military suicide cited in the MPTSR report). One Facebook user responded to a post on the Military with PTSD support group page on October 26, 2014, to express her feelings about SSRIs. She said: "Fluoxetine...made me pure nuts!!! I had to be straight jacketed." There is also a large body of evidence that suggests that SSRIs lead to "worrisome suicidal acts and ideation" (Burstow 2015, p. 316).

Other types of medications commonly prescribed are atypical antipsychotics such as Seroquel, Zyprexa, and Geodon (in combination with SSRIs) and benzodiazepines (also called "anti-anxiety drugs"). The first three can cause weight gain, diabetes, and cardiovascular problems (Hoge 2010, p. 201). I would note, additionally, that many group members on the Military with PTSD Facebook site shared negative experiences with drugs like Seroquel. One user warned: "Seroquel was a really bad choice for me. I became delusional and psychotic"; others stated: "get the heck away from Seroquel" (posted October 25, 2014). It is becoming apparent that benzodiazepines are likely one of the worst choices of drugs when treating military trauma because they have "very detrimental side effects (and) carry a high risk of becoming addictive" according to Hoge (2010, p. 201). A recent study (Guina et al. 2015) also states:

> Benzodiazepines are ineffective for PTSD treatment and prevention, and risks ... outweigh potential short-term benefits. In addition to adverse effects in general populations, benzodiazepines are associated with specific problems in patients with PTSD: worse overall severity, significantly increased risk of developing PTSD with use after recent trauma, worse psychotherapy outcomes, aggression, depression, and substance use. (p. 281)

Many veterans and family members have posted on the Military with PTSD Facebook group about how various combinations of drugs prescribed have negatively impacted their lives. One recent post, soliciting advice from other group members, reads: "My husband a marine vet is diagnosed with severe PTSD. He has been prescribed so many medications to help him cope. He happens to get almost all the severe side affects so has had to stop the meds every time. His psychiatrist is so heartbroken and emotional because she is running out of ways to help him. [*sic*]" (July 12, 2015). This post elicited more than 250 comments. Many of them came from veterans who had also had negative experiences with prescription drug combinations. One veteran wrote: "I also have horrible side effects from the medications the VA has given me. I keep having hallucinations with some and really felt as though I was losing my mind" (July 12).

Another commenter gave advice: "Cut the drugs, my therapist was annoyed and said I was evasive. NOT the truth. I wanted the strength to be the master of my own issues [*sic*]" (July 12). Another woman commented: "My husband has PTSD and for a long time, it was hard to find out what worked for him and his symptoms. Medication did not work for him either. It was like living with a zombie. So we dropped the meds." Another commenter was more forceful with his advice:

> These people (psychiatrists) LOVE to medicate. And they do more harm than good... (They) want only to use extremely potent anti-psychotics...these meds ALWAYS are with side effects—the MAJOR, CAUSING him to appear psychotic. In patient care—well, did that in Phoenix Arizona, twice. DO NOT RECOMMEND THIS. More chances to "practice" psych- medicate him into oblivion, then do anything useful.... Those of us that are veterans would really like to believe the VA will actually help us—sadly, ALL they really want to do is MEDICATE into numbness—NO WAY TO LIVE! [*sic*]

Many others who commented on this particular post suggested moving away from traditional psychiatric treatment altogether. Alternatives that they saw as helpful and so recommended included: acupuncture, reiki, deep breathing, talking to other veterans, exercise, healthy eating, equine therapy, scuba diving, and (the most common suggestion) getting a service dog.

Still—and here we see the extent of the hegemony—many posts reflected a strong faith in the system. One commenter wrote: "I recommend going to an inpatient facility. It helped me after 21 years." Another wrote: "Most importantly he needs to continue his treatment. He CAN NOT HELP YOU if he doesn't help himself." Another wrote: "These prpgrams really work. They really work with veterans putting them through uncomfortable places to show them its okay and they can become comfortable with it. I hope he gets the help he needs" [*sic*]. Other people specified that even though it took them 11–12 times in inpatient programs, "eventually" they were able to give into treatment and start to "recover."

A post on June 27, 2015, garnered a similar reaction of mixed responses from members of the Military with PTSD Facebook group. The post read: "We laid my husband to rest, 6/25 - Ptsd is real and awful. Please get your loved one help." This particular post garnered 3199 "likes," 1142 "shares," and 240 comments. Many of the comments echoed the sentiments expressed by the original poster and linked PTSD to suicide. At least a dozen men and women wrote saying that their own husband/brother/son/ was driven to suicide because of PTSD. Some commenters did offer critiques of the treatment they had received, however. What was noteworthy in these posts is that even those commenters who appear to profoundly distrust psychiatry and the "treatment" they or their loved ones have received, still activate the language of the DSM on a regular basis, and insist that "PTSD is real."

How buy-in like this happens is evident from the tracing done to date. Just look at the figure earlier in the chapter, and it is only too clear why. It also can be seen just by looking at what these site administrators post. For example, an inspirational quote an administrator posted on The Military Minds Facebook site on June 16 shows a photo of a bridge with a caption that reads:

> We all say "we'll cross that bridge when we come to it." Well, it's time. You've arrived. About you and your PTSD, you can continue to procrastinate and stay where you are or you can move forward. Time to break the silence and get moving. We'll shoulder your ruck.

Or a June 17 picture of six soldiers from what appears to be WWI, each holding a rifle. The caption for that photo reads:

> Who misses it? Coming off a morning "cleaning patrol." Regardless of what year it is, it's all the same, for only the technology changes. Same goes for PTSD. It's been around since the beginning, and only the name has changed. Now we have the resources to do something about it. Use 'em.

Such captions and the large number of "likes" they receive from group members indicate that soldiers and veterans are encouraged to bring the idea of PTSD and the concept of the drug cure into their everyday "work"—and indeed, as we have already seen, many do.

Herein lies a further conundrum—and how it is institutionally created, we have already caught a glimpse of.

Concluding Remarks

This chapter has traced how it has come to pass that a fictional disorder "essentially created by committees of doctors sitting around conference tables" (Hoge 2010, p. 6) has gained so much traction in recent years. I have traced how the ruling relations continually associate the idea of PTSD with soldiers' suicides and how the language of the DSM is now regularly activated. This is done not only by the media, the military, and the psychiatric system itself but also by service members, veterans, and those closest to them as they go about their daily lives.

To reinforce the sentiment expressed earlier in this chapter, the tragic irony here is that activating the boss text in this way directly leads to "treatment" that characteristically irreversibly damages those it purports to "help."

References

Boone, K. N. (2011). The paradox of PTSD. *The Wilson Quarterly, 35*(4), 18–22.

Brewster, M. (2013, December 4). Canadian soldier attempts suicide after PTSD ends military career. *The Toronto Star.* Retrieved from http://www.thestar.com/news/canada/2013/12/04/canadian_soldier_attempts_suicide_after_ptsd_ends_military_career.html

Burstow, B. (2005). A critique of post traumatic stress disorder and the DSM. *Journal of Humanistic Psychology, 45*(4), 429–445.

Burstow, B. (2015). Psychiatry and the business of madness: An ethical and epistomological accounting. New York: Palgrave Macmillan.

Campion-Smith, B. (2014a, September 16). Suicide claims more soldiers than those killed by Afghan combat. *The Toronto Star.* Retrieved from: http://www.thestar.com/news/canada/2014/09/16/suicide_claims_more_soldiers_than_those_killed_by_afghan_combat.html

Campion-Smith, B. (2014b, November 25). Canadian vets face long waits for mental health help, auditor says. *The Toronto Star.* Retrieved from: http://www.thestar.com/news/canada/2014/11/25/canadian_veterans_face_long_waits_for_mental_health_help_auditor_says.html

Canadian Soldier Involved in Standoff with Police Dies by Suicide [video file]. (2014, September 16). Retrieved from: http://www.ctvnews.ca/canada/canadian-soldier-involved-in-standoff-with-police-dies-by-suicide-1.2010243

Childress, S. (2015, April 3). What we still don't understand about military suicides. *Frontline.* Retrieved from: http://www.pbs.org/wgbh/pages/frontline/foreign-affairs-defense/what-we-still-dont-understand-about-military-suicides/

Cukor, J., Spitalnick, J., Difede, J, et al. (2009). Emerging treatments for PTSD. *Clinical Psychology Review, 29*, 715-726.

Dao, J., & Lehren, A. W. (2013, May 16). Baffling rise in suicides plagues US military. *The New York Times*. Retrieved from http://www.nytimes.com/2013/05/16/us/baffling-rise-in-suicides-plagues-us-military.html?_r=0

Dreazen, Y. (2014, November 7). Five myths about military suicides. *The Washington Post*. Retrieved from: http://www.washingtonpost.com/opinions/five-myths-about-suicide-in-the-military/2014/11/07/61ceb0aa-637b-11e4-836c-83bc4f26eb67_story.html

Grant, K. (2014, August 11). Post-traumatic stress disorder doubles among Canadian Forces. *The Globe and Mail*. Retrieved from http://www.theglobeandmail.com/news/national/one-in-six-military-members-have-mental-health-problems-statscan-says/article19990160/

Guina, J., Rossetter, S. R., Derhodes, B., Nahhas, R., & Welton, R. (2015). Benzodiazepines for PTSD. *Journal of Psychiatric Practice, 21*(4), 281.

Hale, J. (2015, July 9). Vet to Media: We're not all broken. *Michigan Radio*. Retrieved from: http://michiganradio.org/post/vet-media-were-not-all-broken#stream/0

Herber, A.,& Roux, S. (2015). Military Professional Technical Suicide Review (MPTSR) report. Retrieved from http://www.cimvhr.ca/sghrp_reports/summary.php?ftype=2&tval=Medical%20Professional%20Technical%20Suicide%20Review%20Report

Hoge, C. (2010). *Once a warrior, always a warrior*. Guilford: Lyons Press.

Kime, P. (2015a, April 2). Military study: No link between combat and suicides. *USA Today*.Retrievedfrom:http://www.usatoday.com/story/news/nation/2015/04/02/suicide-troops-veterans-combat-study/70842540/

Kime, P. (2015b, June 17). Senate to VA: End mindless narcotics prescriptions now. *Military Times*. Retrieved from: http://www.militarytimes.com/story/military/benefits/veterans/2015/06/16/tammy-baldwin-legislation-protect-veterans-from-overprescribing-opioids/71262276/

Mackenzie, L. (2014, February 14). Canadian Forces: Holding the line on mental health. *The Globe and Mail*. Retrieved from http://www.theglobeandmail.com/globe-debate/canadian-forces-holding-the-line-on-mental-health/article16892831/

Mental Health and Wellness. Health Canada. Retrieved from http://www.hc-sc.gc.ca/fniah-spnia/promotion/mental/index-eng.php

Mental Health in the Military: Ottawa to Spend $200M over 6 Years (2014, November23).Retrievedfromhttp://www.cbc.ca/news/politics/mental-health-in-the-military-ottawa-to-spend-200m-over-6-years-1.2846166

Military Minds Inc. Retrieved from www.militarymindsinc.com

Monson, C. M., Taft, C. T., & Fredman, S. J. (2009). Military-related PTSD and intimate relationships: From description to theory-driven research and intervention development. *Clinical Psychology Review, 29*, 707–714.

Nazarov, A., Jetly, R., McNeely, H., Kiang, M., Lanius, R., & McKinnon, M. C. (2015). Role of morality in the experience of guilt and shame within the armed forces. *Acta Psychiatrica Scandinavica, 142*, 4–19.

Pearson, C., Zamorsji, M., & Janz, T. (2014) Mental health of the Canadian Armed Forces. *Statistics Canada*. Retrieved from http://www.statcan.gc.ca/pub/82-624-x/2014001/article/14121-eng.htm

Philipps, D. (2015, April 1). Study finds no link between military suicide rate and deployments. *The New York Times*. Retrieved from http://www.nytimes. com/2015/04/02/us/study-finds-no-link-between-military-suicide-rate-and-deployments.html

Post-traumatic Stress Disorder. (n.d.). Department of National Defence website. Retrieved from http://www.forces.gc.ca/en/news/article.page?doc=post-traumatic-stress-disorder/hjlbrhp4

Professional Treatment Overview: Clinician's guide to medications for PTSD. US Department of Veterans Affairs website. http://www.ptsd.va.gov/professional/treatment/overview/clinicians-guide-to-medications-for-ptsd.asp

Sher, J. (2011, March 7). Canadian soldiers in Afghanistan suffer high rate of brain trauma. *The Globe and Mail*. Retrieved from http://www.theglobeandmail.com/news/politics/canadian-soldiers-in-afghanistan-suffer-high-rate-of-brain-trauma/article569601/War/

Smith, D. (1983). No one commits suicide: Textual analysis of ideological practices. *Human Studies, 6*(1), *309–359*.

Smith, D. (2005). *Institutional ethnography: A sociology for people*. New York: Altamira Press.

Smith, D. (2006). *Institutional ethnography as practice*. New York: Rowman & Littlefield Publishers, Inc.

Soldier Suicides: "National Tragedy" Demands Action, Vets Say. (2013, December 5). *The Toronto Star*. Retrieved from http://www.thestar.com/news/canada/2013/12/05/soldier_suicides_national_tragedy_demands_action_vets_say.html

Suicide and Suicide Prevention in the Canadian Armed Forces. Canadian Armed Forces website. Retrieved from http://www.forces.gc.ca/en/news/article.page?doc=suicide-and-suicide-prevention-in-the-canadian-armed-forces/hgq87xvu#anc2

Tucker, E. (2014, January 20). Timeline: Recent soldier suicides in Canada's military. *Global News*. Retrieved from http://globalnews.ca/news/1094652/timeline-recent-soldier-suicides-in-canadas-military/

Waters, S. (2006). *Hero book: An illustrated memoir*. Toronto: Cumulus Press.

CHAPTER 8

The Caring Professions, Not So Caring?: An Analysis of Bullying and Emotional Distress in the Academy

Jemma Tosh and Sarah Golightley

In this chapter we analyze two case studies of bullying at United Kingdom (UK) universities, one involving a student of social work and another of a faculty member in a psychology department. The initial disjuncture in one case study occurred when a victim of bullying was labeled as "mentally ill," and the second was when someone was bullied because of a label of "mental illness." These two similar but opposing disjunctures offer an opportunity for comparative analysis. This includes an investigation of the processes and discourses at play within the broader context of UK higher education and constructions of bullying and emotional distress.

A combination of institutional ethnography (IE) (Smith 1986, 2005) and discourse analysis (Burman 2004; Ian Parker 2013, 2014) is used to analyze these experiences and related texts (e.g., university policy documents). The analysis delineates how the reporting of bullying and harassment was reframed as "incompetency" and "emotional vulnerability." The focus is on how people who are perceived or labeled as having a "mental illness" have been further victimized and pathologized by academic institutions, and how this connects to homophobia, transphobia, ableism, and those who take a critical stance against psychiatry.

The context of UK higher education has changed dramatically within a political and economic context of austerity, to include controversial increases in tuition fees, restructuring of support for students, as well as changes in how universities

J. Tosh (✉)
Simon Fraser University, Burnaby, Canada
e-mail: jemma_tosh@sfu.ca

S. Golightley
Social Work, University of Edinburgh, Edinburgh, Scotland, UK

© The Editor(s) (if applicable) and The Author(s) 2016
B. Burstow (ed.), *Psychiatry Interrogated*,
DOI 10.1007/978-3-319-41174-3_8

are assessed and funded (Deem 1998; Deem et al. 2007; Grimshaw and Rubery 2012; Levidow 2002). These transformations have resulted in notable changes in the working culture of UK universities, particularly in relation to unstable employment; increased pressure on staff to "publish, not perish"; and documented bullying, harassment, violence, and emotional distress such as depression, anxiety, and suicidal ideation (Academics Anonymous 2014; Farley and Sprigg 2014; Jameson 2012; Keashly and Neuman 2010; Khoo 2010).

The current project examines the negative impacts of such changes on staff and student well-being by qualitatively analyzing two case studies of bullying at UK universities. We also analyze the role of sanism (Birnbaum 1960; Perlin 2006) in the victimization of these two individuals, and interrogate the use of psychiatric labels to further justify bullying and abuse. These case studies are from the perspective of both faculty and student, in addition to examining the role of departments that center on issues related to emotional distress: social work and psychology.

SOCIAL WORK

Regulation of social work students in England and Wales began in 2005; it was put in place by the General Social Care Council (GSCC), which required prospective and current students to declare whether they had experienced a "serious mental health problem" (Collins 2006, p. 451). This was tied to understandings of "risk," which have been a long-standing and central issue within the profession, because of several high-profile cases of children who died while known to social work services and where malpractice was said to have occurred (Sin and Fong 2009). These stories were part of a broader media sensationalism (and scapegoating) that depicted social work professionals as inadequate at protecting those deemed "vulnerable" (Webb 2006).

Following disclosure of a "mental health problem," prospective students are then subject to a formal investigation of their "fitness to practice," a procedure that was criticized by the Disability Rights Commission in 2007, which recommended that the process be revoked (Beresford and Boxall 2012, p. 158). Beresford and Boxall, social work academics who have spoken openly of their experiences of mental distress, described their experience as follows:

> At several meetings (including a taskforce consultation in May 2009) where social work practice assessors have argued strenuously that students with mental health difficulties should be "screened out" at the application stage and not accepted onto courses of social work education. (p. 158)

This places the social work applicant or student in a tricky position in declaring an experience of emotional distress or dis/ability. On the one hand, declaration provides rights under the Equality Act of 2010 to "reasonable adjustments" and protection against harassment on the grounds of "mental health" or disability (Spandler and Anderson 2015). On the other hand, it also increases the likelihood of experiencing discrimination, bullying, or harassment (Corrigan et al. 2004; Thornicroft 2006).

More recent applications do not require a person to disclose health history or status unless it is deemed to "impinge" on their ability to carry out social work duties or to pose a "risk" to others. Nevertheless, applicants must still agree that staff from the course are allowed to inquire with their general practitioner (GP) or other medical professionals about their suitability for the course (Holmstrom et al. 2014). This medical approach to disability considers the student or applicant to embody an individualized *lacking* and, subsequently, the ability to "manage" this "absence" is subject to scrutiny rather than the educational institution or the discipline itself (Sin and Fong 2009).

Overt exclusions, such as those described by Beresford and Boxall (2012), are rarely acknowledged publicly in the social work profession. Still, those experiencing emotional distress are often all too aware of the barriers to access and the inadequacy of support (Reid and Poole 2013). Students report feeling excluded from class discussions, pathologized by course materials, and as a result, self-censor their histories of emotional distress (Beresford and Boxall 2012; Collins 2006). This is not surprising given the way such students are viewed: "Instead of being understood as having a recognized disability, students were viewed as needy, difficult, and unworthy of what was perceived as special treatment" in social work education (Reid and Poole 2013, p. 217). However, if prospective or current students do not declare their health history in full and it is discovered later, it can be considered a "failure to disclose" and be subject to investigation that can result in them being excluded from training (Currer 2009).

Such social work policies of exclusion exist alongside policies that require all social work courses to have service user involvement components (Beresford and Boxall 2012). Nevertheless, there is a false divide between social work academic, student, and service user. In Canada, Poole et al. (2012) observe that:

> Practices have often led to a divisive "us" and "them" mentality in social work where "we," the rational, well, social work practitioners decide on and distance ourselves from "them," the irrational, "ill" users of "mental health" and social work services (who may also want to be social work students). (p. 24)

This has led critics to assert that service user language has been appropriated for the purposes of masking oppressive practice, and that service user involvement only allows for minimal input. Such critics have concluded that these tokenistic gestures fail to challenge pervasive institutional sanism and albeism (Barnes and Cotterell 2011; Beresford and Boxall 2012).

PSYCHOLOGY

Although many psychologists differentiate (or distance) themselves from psychiatry, biomedical approaches and psychiatric diagnoses predominate within the discipline (Cheshire and Pilgrim 2004; Pilgrim 2007). Psychology's foundation is based on the study and promotion of a "norm," one that is measured and analyzed (Rose 1979). Quantitative analyses that focus on statistics, means, and measurement remain the principal research methods taught in psychology training courses (Fine 2007; Forrester and Koutsopoulou 2008; Hanson and Rapley 2008; Harper et al. 2008). Thus, campaigns against pathologization are closely tied to movements toward the diversification of research methods within psychology; this is because statistical concepts are the very basis from which students learn to reduce human complexity to quantifiable data for the purposes of comparison to a constructed "norm" with "deviations" positioned as Other/"abnormal" from the outset. The hostility and difficulties documented by those engaging in active challenges to the predominance of quantitative/statistical methods and theory within psychology (Burman 1997; Luttrell 2005; Povee and Roberts 2014) illustrate the importance still given to these problematic concepts within the discipline, as well as the resistance to acknowledging psychology's role in the perpetuation of oppression (Tosh 2016).

Burman (1997) draws on the infamous "mind the gap" instruction from the London underground transport system as a way of conceptualizing the disagreement within psychology regarding those approaches that analyze language with those that focus on statistics (i.e., qualitative vs. quantitative research). She argues that the underlying philosophical positions of these qualitative methods—i.e., social constructionism and relativism, see Burr (2015) and Parker (1998)—are incompatible with statistical approaches and that this distinction is an important one to preserve (as do others; see Luttrell 2005). This disparity and long-standing disagreement within the profession has led to qualitative methods having a rather "bad reputation," being undervalued as a method, and often being seen as not "scientific enough" by both staff and students (Hanson and Rapley 2008; Harper et al. 2008; Povee and Roberts 2014; Tosh et al. 2014).

Consequently, there are many barriers to teaching qualitative methods, and obstacles for students to overcome if they are to pursue qualitative research. These can include: a lack of departmental support and, in some cases, hostility and stigma (Harper 2012; Harper et al. 2008; Povee and Roberts 2014; Shaw et al. 2008; Tosh et al. 2014). Shaw et al. (2008) argue that the underlying devaluation of qualitative methods is a result of the relationship between psychology and the natural sciences (e.g., biology), and that this contributes to a context of derision and exclusion. From the student's perspective, calls for more support from staff and peers, as well as an end to the ridiculing of staff and students who employ qualitative methods, are a standard feature of evaluations, feedback, and research in this area (Harper et al. 2008; Povee and Roberts 2014; Tosh et al. 2014).

Like social work, there is often an assumption that those studying or working within psychology are separate from the people being studied. In my work supporting students (labeled) with "mental health problems," this often was an issue discussed: How lectures and teaching materials framed "normal" development in ways that failed to represent them or their life experience, and that they could only relate to the experiences or descriptions of those positioned as "abnormal." For some, it was too much to bear, and they chose to step away from the profession.

There can be similar issues for lecturers required to teach "core" content that can be sexist, homophobic, and transphobic (Ansara and Hegarty 2012; Henwood 1994; Phillips and Fischer 1998; Ellis et al. 2003; Voss and Gannon 1978). For example, comparisons of "sex differences" are common in the teaching of research methods, as is the teaching of evolutionary theories of "mating behaviors" based on sexist and heteronormative ideals (Gannon 2002; Symons 2013). Within psychology transgender individuals are often framed as "perverse" or "mentally ill" when their gender identity goes against that assigned or assumed by medics (Ansara and Hegarty 2012). This is in addition to its problematic framing (or absence) of issues related to racism and ableism (Campbell 2009; Phoenix 1994). Such a pathologizing foundation can make for a difficult work environment for those who fail to live up to this narrowly constructed concept of "normalcy."

METHODOLOGY

As stated earlier, we are employing a case study approach. One case study is about a postgraduate student who was bullied within a UK university social work department during her studies. The second involves the victimization of a faculty member in a UK university psychology department. Both are analyzed using IE (Smith 1986, 2005) and discourse analysis (Parker 2013, 2014; Burman 2004). We also draw on feminist, poststructuralist theory (Weedon 1996) and critical intersectionality theory (Cole 2009; Crenshaw 1991). Therefore, we examine how these occurrences of bullying came to be and how the bullying and harassment were constructed, and we consider intersecting oppressions related to gender and sexuality.

Another aspect of the project is the analysis of sanism—that is, social inequality or oppression based on a diagnosis of "mental illness," according to Birnbaum (1960) and Perlin (2006)—and the questioning of the label of "mental illness" in line with our prior research work (Tosh 2011, 2013, 2015). We bring to this analysis our experience as qualified practitioners, academics within the caring professions, and/or personal experiences of emotional distress. Thus, the analysis includes how an individual was labeled as "mentally ill" in response to the bullying, and how another was bullied following a label of "mental illness." The examination of the *misuse* of such labels and the victimization they can attract forms a key basis of the research inquiry. Our analysis shows how applying these labels can form part of a wider context of bullying and harassment, within a culture where sanism functions.

ESTHER

Esther (pseudonym) was a master's (MA) student in a social work program at an English university. She stated that she had experienced depression for most of her life. When she applied to study social work, she was asked to disclose whether she had any diagnoses in the last five years and whether she had been taking any medication, thus activating "boss texts" related to professional regulation and assessment of risk. Esther was hesitant to disclose and chose not to detail her health history on the declaration form; she stated that she was not technically required to disclose because her diagnosis was more than five years ago and she was not on medication.

Once in the course, Esther felt that she did not fit in with the ethos of the classroom. She described herself as an outspoken queer woman who would challenge the assumptions and politics of her classmates as well as the teachers. Esther described "othering" language used in the course that she considered to be marginalizing and reductive:

> The course would get people to come in for "Service User Involvement" as if they are the separate group and I'm sitting in class every day and I have experiences of having social workers, I have perspectives … obviously not everyone [with these experiences] will be willing to talk about it, but I was willing to talk.

Esther described wanting to challenge the "othering" language by being open about her experience of mental distress. She also wanted to apply for the Disabled Student's Allowance (DSA), which would enable her to access provisions of "reasonable adjustments" (Equality and Human Rights Commission 2015).

To claim DSA provisions Esther had to register as a disabled student at the support unit at her university. She filled in a form explaining that she had been diagnosed with depression and that she was a student in the social work course. She was then required to meet with a "mental health" advisor to discuss her "condition" and what reasonable adjustments she would need. In line with university policy, the support unit's website outlined that this discussion would be confidential.

The disjuncture occurred when the "mental health" advisor explained to Esther at the end of the meeting that because she had disclosed a "mental health problem," he would need to inform her teacher that their meeting would not be confidential because social work students are covered by different policies relating to their study. Therefore, the confidentiality statement within the context of the support unit was not the boss text being activated; instead it was the policies and regulations of social work professionals and those in training.

This change in approach or policy was stated to be because of the potential "risks" of Esther having a perceived "undeclared health condition." Esther stated that she was given the option of telling the teacher about her "depression"—or the advisor would do it for her. Esther opted to be the one to tell. She also asked the teacher how to lay a complaint against the advisor as she felt that being treated as "risky" was unfounded and that she had not been appropriately informed about her confidentiality rights, or lack thereof, at the beginning of the meeting. Esther stated:

> People [in the social work course] spoke like "this is what people with mental health problems are like, this is how [to] deal with them and interact with them" … there seemed a barrier to what people were able to disclose about themselves … the fact that nobody was talking [about their own experiences] was troubling.

The teacher then informed the course convener who subsequently told a staff member at Esther's course placement (i.e., her student internship). Esther recalled receiving an email stating that she had to attend an "emergency meeting" to discuss what was termed a "failure to disclose" her health history. Esther described the meeting as follows:

> [I said] What do you mean failure to disclose? … this approach is ableist and contradictory to anti-oppressive social work … you are making it less accessible for people with mental health problems and all of those associated with higher rates of mental health problems, such as queers and people of color. … [T]here is silence about mental health because people are afraid of responses like this [the emergency meeting]. … It should be my choice what I share, it is not "hiding" anything, it is protective.

Esther decided to speak to the student newspaper to describe her experience of discrimination during her course. She believed that going public with her story was more likely to affect change than making a formal complaint. Once the news article was published (anonymously), the course convener called another "emergency meeting" to discuss details about Esther potentially being "kicked off the course" for "bringing the profession into disrepute," activating additional policies regarding student conduct and public information about the university and its reputation.

The British Association of Social Workers (BASW) "Code of Ethics" (2014) principles include challenging discrimination, challenging unjust policies and practices, as well as recognizing diversity (p. 9). It further states that social workers should confront contravention of human rights and be prepared to be a whistle-blower: "Social workers should be prepared to report bad practice using all available channels including complaints procedures and if necessary use public interest disclosure legislation and whistleblowing guidelines" (BASW 2014, p. 14). The Code of Ethics, however, also stipulates that social workers are supposed to "uphold the reputation" and not "bring the profession into disrepute" (p. 10). Depending on which part of the text is activated, we can see that the same code can be used selectively against people who speak up, or in support of people who speak up at injustice within social work (Figure 8.1).

Following the publication of the anonymous article, the social work department refused a second practice placement to which it had initially agreed. They cited that her "disability" required her to have a placement closer to campus in case she needed support; however, while they were activating university texts regarding support for disabled students, this was contrary to Esther's experience, as being close to the university was never assessed as one of her support needs. Ultimately, she was not given the placement she had initially agreed to and soon apprehensions were expressed about her new placement.

Esther described raising several concerns about her placement, including the lack of supervision and being assigned work that was not suitable for students. She also raised questions about institutional practice when she found notes

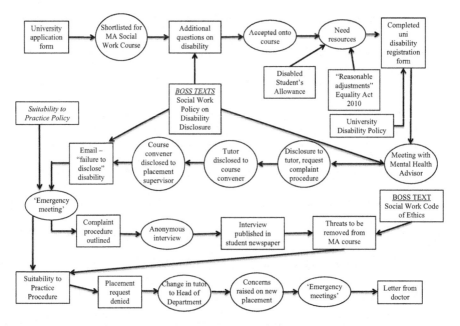

Figure 8.1   Sanism in social work education

that a woman with a "traveler background" with "mental health problems" had been sterilized without a record of consent. This prompted further "emergency meetings" where Esther was framed as having "problems with authority," being "resistant to work," feeling "insecure," and being "full of self-doubt" about her ability to do her work. Feedback from the service users and from colleagues was positive and her grades were above average, so the criticisms did not fit with a "reality check" from others. If she challenged these assumptions it would be seen as confirmation of her problems with authority and even small, seemingly irrelevant things were pathologized as signs of emotional issues.

Esther noted that her placement supervisors and teachers interpreted everything she did as wrong. Her desk was moved away from her supportive colleagues and placed next to her supervisor's, who scrutinized her closely. She said she was "trying to keep my head down and get on with things"; however, even when she followed the advice of her supervisors, they would later criticize her for having done so. It became clear to Esther that she was being prevented from completing a successful placement. Esther elaborated, explaining:

> She [the placement supervisor] said, "I have a suggestion for you, how would you feel if I became your only assessor?" … I said that I would feel bad ending supervision with the other assessor. … [S]he replied saying, "if you want to pass, you need to do what's best for you and this is what I recommend." She later [in a meeting with the university] said to me that she thought I "lacked empathy" for

choosing to get rid of the other assessor. At this point I was just in tears, think-ing, "I can't believe how manipulative this is," and my [university] tutor who I had also gone to before was not sticking up for me ... I called them out on it, I said, "You both advised me on this" ... then this is where "problems of authority" came out again. ... [T]he conclusion of that meeting was the only way I could continue the placement would be if I were willing to talk to the placement asses-sor about my childhood and "my problems."

Esther, realizing she was in a no-win situation, ended the placement without failing by activating health-related policies and procedures. She went to her GP saying: "This is bad for my health, I need to stop." She was given a supporting letter and went back to the university's Suitability to Practice Assessor. Esther was allowed to defer and start a new placement the following year.

OLIVIA

The disjuncture for the second case study occurred when a faculty member of a university psychology department, Olivia (pseudonym), returned to work after a short period of illness. On her return, she was accused of feigning her illness based on, what her line manager termed, "gossip" within the department. This speculation was attributed to the fact that Olivia had an impending deadline related to her work. She was accused of taking sick leave to avoid her depart-mental responsibilities and to pursue her own research.

The reasons given for her accusation were that she was viewed as a particu-larly motivated researcher; Olivia stated:

It really took the wind out of me. I was so shocked. It never even occurred to me that I would be accused of such a thing. I just burst into tears. All I could think of was, what a horrible thing to think of me ... to think that I was that kind of person. ... At the same time, it explained a lot. I thought I was paranoid in the way that people were looking at me, and talking, then going silent when I entered a room or got close. I did become very socially anxious.

This represents a disjuncture as it was not only distressing to be accused in this way but also it was an unusual occurrence and a departure from standard departmental behavior and, indeed, boss texts. For instance, as it was within Olivia's job description as a lecturer to pursue research, and the university was leading up to an important and soon to occur external research assessment, being a "motivated" researcher did not single Olivia out from her departmen-tal peers. Many, if not most, of her colleagues would be rigorously pursuing research and research deadlines at this same time. Also, other colleagues had been off sick.

Therefore, this act of accusing Olivia of lying about her illness took a stark departure from the "norms" of the department, from both standard job descrip-tions and "invisible" boss texts that function alongside them—for example, believing staff when they state they are unwell when there is no evidence to the contrary. It also showed discriminatory behavior because Olivia was treated differently for doing something that most individuals in academia do (i.e., pursue research).

In addition, then, to failing to activate invisible boss texts within the department, there was a failure to activate relevant texts such as university policy documents. For example, Olivia reported to her line manager her experiences of bullying and harassment, including ongoing "gossip"; spreading of "malicious rumors," threats, and verbal abuse; and shouting (in private and in front of staff and students), resulting in public humiliation. Furthermore, colleagues and senior members of staff took away her responsibilities when she was capable of completing the work and excluded her from team events and meetings, while senior members of the staff also pressured her to participate in social groups that were actively bullying her.

All of these were listed in the university's policy as examples of "bullying" and "harassment." Nevertheless, her complaint was never taken forward, despite it being required for her line manager to report such incidents to human resources and to monitor the situation. Instead, her experience was reframed as a problem with "workload" followed by accusations of inexperience, regardless of evidence to the contrary— initially, Olivia had been told that she was hired specifically for her experience in qualitative research and teaching.

As the bullying continued, behavior of colleagues and senior staff moved even further away from the job description. Olivia was instructed to stop all research activity. Then she was prevented from doing any teaching within the department. These were the two main aspects of her job as a lecturer and as an academic in a university department. She was instead instructed to spend her time marking assignments for her colleagues and "socializing" in the department. Olivia was highly monitored in this aspect, discouraged from working in her office or working independently, and required to check in with two senior members of the staff daily on her marking progress: "I was moved closer to senior members of staff, my office I mean. I was told this was so that they could 'keep an eye on me.'"

These unusual requests, that contradicted the job description document, represented an activation of another boss text, but one that was not relevant to this situation: the university policy on staff with "mental health problems." Therefore, while the university policy on bullying and harassment was not activated, despite a report of bullying and harassment, and the invisible boss text of appropriate supportive behavior when a staff member returned to work was not activated, the policy on "mental illness" *was* activated. This was in terms of making "reasonable adjustments," despite the staff member not having a formal diagnosis.

The report of bullying—of victimization within the department by colleagues (and senior staff members)—was reframed as an internal pathology within Olivia, as a "nervous breakdown" and "anxiety." Correspondingly, the restrictions on her work were framed as a consequence of her fragility and incompetence. Reports from students that they were uncomfortable with staff "speaking badly behind [her] back," "making fun of [her] in lectures," and fears that "[she] would lose [her] job" were reframed as a "workload issue." The narrative that Olivia had a "breakdown" because of her "anxiety" was so dominant that contradictory evidence was ignored or framed as further "lies" and thus used as more evidence of her "mental health problem." For example, Olivia stated:

> I couldn't believe it when I heard [a colleague] say that I deserved all the marking I was being given because I had dropped the ball on my teaching. When I asked what she meant, she explained that the whole department had been told (in a team meeting) that I hadn't prepared any teaching materials and that's why I pretended to be sick. This was outrageous! Not only had I prepared the materials over a year in advance, but I had a sick note from the doctor explaining that I was off sick due to work-related stress, because of the bullying. My line manager knew this, and chose to lie to the department, but no one would believe me.

This breached further university policy (as well as legal texts regarding slander), but it showed that policies on confidentiality were also not being activated despite being relevant to the situation. Olivia commented that on several occasions she thought she was "going mad" because colleagues would stare at her and discuss private details about her life, but she had no idea how they knew such information. She later found out that colleagues had been sharing information from her private social media account and that her line manager regularly updated the team in meetings about private life events (e.g., ill health of a relative) without her knowledge or consent.

This was framed as "helping" and "supporting" Olivia, but resulted in her private life being the content of departmental "gossip" that was used to support constructions of her as "weak," "vulnerable," and ultimately, incapable of doing her job. Excluding Olivia from meetings helped to exacerbate this. She was instructed not to attend staff meetings, and thus was unable to defend herself from accusations or state that the information was private. About this Olivia said:

> I remember walking down the hallway, trying my best just to keep it together. I can't describe how it feels, to walk around feeling like all eyes are on you. ... Then one of the [senior members of staff] approached me and asked how my mother was doing. I nearly threw up. My first thought was that I was trying not to think about her being ill when I was at work, because it was upsetting. My second thought was, how the hell do you know?

It also fueled feelings of monitoring, that every aspect of her life (and work) was scrutinized in unpredictable ways. For example, after publishing a paper that described a successful teaching intervention around qualitative methods and gender, Olivia was called into her line manager's office and "screamed at for over an hour." Accused of making the department look bad, Olivia was told that she "would be fired," would "never work in the discipline again" because "academia is a small world." This escalated, according to Olivia, to the manager saying: "[E]veryone in the department is so angry at this. You should avoid everyone because I'm not sure what they will do. They are furious with you and can't wait for you to leave." Again, this was in direct contrast to numerous boss texts that could/should have been activated, such as bullying and harassment, and numerous texts related to "respect" within the workplace. Olivia commented that it was this framing of the responses as "the whole department" that had such an effect on her:

> I didn't know who was friend or foe, or who to even approach. I had already been assaulted in my office (by a student who commented that I didn't have the support of my colleagues) and genuinely feared that this "furious" "mob" of colleagues would physically hurt me. It sounds absurd, but that's what I was told. I found out later, just before I left, that the whole thing had been a lie, and it was only really three people. I wish I had known at the time and told people what was happening to me.

Ironically, while Olivia was labeled as "mentally ill," which was then used as justification for further victimization and discrimination, the bullying itself caused severe emotional distress—distress that was ignored, according to Olivia:

> Everyone made out that they were so supportive of my anxiety and breakdown, y'know, "oh, poor you, if we ask you to do anything, you'll break." Yet, when I cried in my office, and I mean cried, that kind of crying you do when you can't stop, and you can't breathe, and you sob, big loud sobs that no matter how hard you try, you can't suppress—nothing. They heard, they listened, they did not help. I would self-harm in my office, and I contemplated suicide. The only thing that got me through it, were my students. God how I loved my students! They knew something was up, and they were the ones who supported me, not the psychologists who are supposed to be experts in "mental health," not even those who researched bullying! If you want empathy in academia, go to your students. They will keep you alive, and hopeful.

Olivia also noted how the students were central to her gaining a "truthful" understanding of the situation. While rumors and gossip filled the department, students reported what was being said (to Olivia, not the university) and also alluded to possible motives of those harassing her:

> I heard all kinds of horror stories from students, upset that they were being told in lectures that "bisexuality is just a phase in adolescence" and that transgender people have a "brain disease," then I thought, oh crap. If that's what they think, and that's the kind of hostility that I'm up against, then it's probably impacting on this whole situation.

Olivia described feeling "pushed out" of the profession for challenging the way it views and understands gender and sexuality. She had taken a stand in the department, and profession, against the pathologization of gender and sexual minorities and felt that the problematic views of her colleagues were one reason that she had been targeted in this way.

This coincides with the acknowledgment of homophobia and heteronormative assumptions within psychology (Ellis et al. 2003), as well as the increasing documentation of cisgenderism—the ideology that invalidates or pathologizes self-designated genders that contrast with external designations, according to Ansara and Hegarty (2012, p. 1)—and transphobia within the profession (see more generally, Ansara and Hegarty 2012). This is not surprising, perhaps, because of the long history of psychology and psychiatry in the pathologization and "treatment" of homosexual and transgender people (Tosh 2015, 2016).

Olivia stated at length that the other reason for the bullying was because of her role as departmental lead on qualitative research:

> It was so ridiculous. You had some people in the department stating that I was the "expert" and others who treated me like an inexperienced child. I was asked to redesign the qualitative teaching in the whole department, they even asked for specific methods to cover, when I did what they asked, I mean, I jumped through every hoop, they turned on me at the last minute. With less than 24 hours before my first qualitative lecture, they were like, "Oh, no, we don't want this." I showed them emails from over 12 months ago where they had seen all the materials and plans and replied saying it looked "great" and they "couldn't wait" and that students would "love it," to when the bullying started and these emails started to say "this won't work." "You're going to screw it up," I broke down when I was asked to redesign the teaching—the whole thing, assignments, exams, lectures, seminars, everything, in less than 12 hours. I said it was impossible, but my line manager told me to do it. I stopped breathing. I was crouched on the floor of my office and the room began to spin. I thought to myself, this job isn't worth dying over. I went straight to my GP and told him everything.

Not only does this quote illustrate the harm caused by bullying and harassment within the profession of psychology, but it also shows again how actions of colleagues moved away from boss texts.

For example, the British Psychological Society (BPS) requirements for the Graduate Basis for Chartership (GBC), where qualified individuals become chartered psychologists, state that qualitative methodologies have to be included in psychology teaching, and the subject benchmark statement for psychology states that "new developments" in qualitative research should be incorporated into undergraduate teaching (Quality Assurance Agency for Higher Education 2010, p. 3). Yet, Olivia was prevented from implementing an updated qualitative program that would reflect both of these requirements.

Olivia stated that she felt she had been targeted for her perceived gender identity and sexual orientation, despite never stating either to colleagues or the university, but suspected as well that the strong position she took with respect to research was enough for her to be targeted in this way. She also stated that the hostility that she experienced for trying to implement qualitative teaching in the psychology course, which moved away from quantitative paradigms and challenged pathologizing approaches, was far beyond what she had expected; Olivia elaborated:

I knew that it would be difficult, I mean, I had been using qualitative methods since I was a student, during my PhD and published on the method—so I was used to ridicule, people who just thought it was a load of rubbish, or professional disagreement. But this was way beyond that; this was targeted, ganging up, emotionally abusive, violent even. I went from happy and confident, to confused and suicidal within a matter of months. Since leaving, though, I have heard stories from so many colleagues. The scariest thing is that I'm not the only one. So many others are suffering in their offices, in silence, thinking there is something wrong with them.

In standing up against the profession and in campaigning for change, once she was labeled as "mentally ill," her "voice was taken from [her]." Olivia said that ultimately, "[i]t forced me out. I quit. What else could I do?"

Concluding Remarks

These two case studies illustrate how labels of "mental illness" can be used to silence those who speak out against oppression and pathologization within those professions where such interventions are sorely needed. In one case, violence and bullying was dismissed, ignored, and perpetuated by labeling the victim as "mentally ill." In doing so, her accusations of bullying and her competency regarding her job became discredited and disbelieved. Her actions and words were constantly interpreted and viewed through the lens of sanism and used as further justification for abuse.

In the other case, the label of "mental illness" was framed as a "danger" and a "risk" in addition to a "vulnerability." However, rather than provide the assistance that was initially requested, her label of mental illness was used in attempts to disrupt her training, much like how Olivia was "pushed out" of her job. This, in addition to the increased surveillance in both cases, shows how "reasonable adjustments" manifested as *restrictions* framed within a discourse of "help" and doing what was "best" for those with a "mental illness."

This coincides with research that suggests people who are perceived as "outsiders" are often the target of bullying (Sedivy-Benton et al. 2015). This "otherness" can be construed because of a person being a new staff member, having different political or social attitudes, being high achieving, revealing their sexuality or gender identity, or for a myriad of other reasons. In these situations, policies do not protect victims, as they can fail to be activated, or are used selectively to either support or silence those who speak out. As others have observed, including Sedivy-Benton et al. (2015):

[The bullies] held all of the power. ... They were not really supervised by the Dean and held accountable, and the program had such convoluted procedures they would interpret arbitrarily and then do whatever they wanted ... procedures were not followed, even though there were protocols and procedures. There were no consequence[s] for not following policy and procedures. (p. 39)

It also is important to note that, in both cases, getting documented evidence from someone external to the university (their GPs) activated boss texts within a context where others failed to activate relevant procedures such as bullying and harassment reporting. For Olivia this resulted in her not having to complete an impossible task (i.e., redesigning her teaching in a short period of time) and for Esther, her ability to delay completion of her course. Therefore, even though bullying and power hierarchies impeded their ability to activate certain procedures, or to ensure that those procedures were carried out in nonoppressive ways, activating texts from outside of the academy enabled protection and possible avenues to challenge and prevent further victimization.

Sanism, then, functions to silence those who speak out, those who do not fit the "norm" promoted by psychology, psychiatry, and social work. Conformity to the constructed "norm" of psychology and psychiatry acts as an invisible boss text that is activated within teaching departments, whereby those who speak out against it or do not fit within its narrow definition of "normal" become victims of a process of humiliation, intimidation, and abuse. The norm maintains the power hierarchies in place by forcing out those who would challenge it, undermine it, and change it.

References

Academics Anonymous. (2014). Bullying in academia: "Professors are supposed to be stressed! That's the job." Retrieved July 15, 2015, from http://www.theguardian.com/higher-education-network/blog/2014/oct/24/bullying-academia-universities-stress-support

Ansara, G., & Hegarty, P. (2012). Cisgenderism in psychology: Pathologising and misgendering children from 1999 to 2008. *Psychology & Sexuality, 3*, 137–160.

Barnes, M., & Cotterell, P. (Eds.) (2011). *Critical perspectives on user involvement.* Bristol: Policy Press.

Beresford, P., & Boxall, K. (2012). Service users, social work education and knowledge for social work practice. *Social Work Education, 31*, 155–167.

Birnbaum, M. (1960). The right to treatment. *American Bar Association Journal, 46*, 499–505.

British Association of Social Workers. (2014). Code of Ethics for social work: Statement of principles. Retrieved June 10, 2015, from www.basw.co.uk/codeofethics

Burman, E. (1997). Minding the gap: Positivism, psychology, and the politics of qualitative methods. *Journal of Social Issues, 53*, 785–801.

Burman, E. (2004). Discourse analysis means analysing discourse: Some comments on Antaki, Billig, Edwards and Potter "Discourse analysis means doing analysis: A critique of six analytic shortcomings." *Discourse Analysis Online, 1.* Retrieved from http://extra.shu.ac.uk/daol/articles/open/2003/003/burman2003003-paper.html

Burr, V. (2015). *Social constructionism.* London: Routledge.

Campbell, F. K. (2009). *Contours of ableism: The production of disability and abledness.* Basingstoke: Palgrave Macmillan.

Cheshire, K., & Pilgrim, D. (2004). *A short introduction to clinical psychology.* London: SAGE Publications.

Cole, E. R. (2009). Intersectionality and research in psychology. *American Psychologist, 64*, 170–180.

Collins, S. (2006). Mental health difficulties and the support needs of social work students: Dilemmas, tensions and contradictions. *Social Work Education, 2*, 446–460.

Corrigan, P. W., Markowitz, F. E., & Watson, A. C. (2004). Structural levels of mental illness stigma and discrimination. *Schizophrenia Bulletin, 30*, 481–491.

Crenshaw, K. (1991). Mapping the margins: Intersectionality, identity politics, and violence against women of color. *Stanford Law Review, 43*, 1241–1299.

Currer, C. (2009). Assessing student social workers' professional suitability: Comparing university procedures in England. *British Journal of Social Work, 39*, 1481–1498.

Deem, R. (1998). "New managerialism" and higher education: The management of performances and cultures in universities in the United Kingdom. *International Studies in Sociology of Education, 8*, 47–70.

Deem, R., Hillyard, S., & Reed, M. (2007). *Knowledge, higher education, and the new managerialism: The changing management of UK universities.* Oxford: Oxford University Press.

Ellis, S., Kitzinger, C., & Wilkinson, S. (2003). Attitudes towards lesbians and gay men and support for lesbian and gay human rights among psychology students. *Journal of Homosexuality, 44*(1), 121–138.

Equality and Human Rights Commission. (2015). What are reasonable adjustments? Equality and Human Rights Commission. Retrieved July 13, 2015, from http://www.equalityhumanrights.com/private-and-public-sector-guidance/education-providers/higher-education-providers-guidance/key-concepts/what-discrimination/reasonable-adjustments

Farley, S., and Sprigg, C. (2014). Culture of cruelty: Why bullying thrives in higher education. Retrieved April 7, 2015 from http://www.theguardian.com/higher-education-network/blog/2014/nov/03/why-bullying-thrives-higher-education

Fine, M. (2007). Expanding the methodological imagination. *The Counseling Psychologist, 35*, 459–473.

Forrester, M. A., & Koutsopoulou, G. Z. (2008). Providing resources for enhancing the teaching of qualitative methods at the undergraduate level: Current practices and the work of the HEA Psychology Network Group. *Qualitative Research in Psychology, 5*, 173–178.

Gannon, L. (2002). A critique of evolutionary psychology. *Psychology, Evolution & Gender, 4*, 173–218.

Grimshaw, D., & Rubery, J. (2012). The end of the UK's liberal collectivist social model? The implications of the coalition government's policy during the austerity crisis. *Cambridge Journal of Economics, 36*, 105–126.

Hanson, S., & Rapley, M. (2008). Editorial: Special issue of qualitative research in psychology on "teaching qualitative methods.". *Qualitative Research in Psychology, 5*, 171–172.

Harper, D. (2012). Surveying qualitative research teaching on British clinical psychology training programmes 1992-2006: A changing relationship? *Qualitative Research in Psychology, 9*, 5–12.

Harper, D., O'Connor, J., Self, P., & Stevens, P. (2008). Learning to use discourse analysis on a professional psychology training programme: Accounts of supervisees and a supervisor. *Qualitative Research in Psychology, 5*, 192–213.

Henwood, K. L. (1994). Resisting racism and sexism in academic psychology: A personal/political view. *Feminism & Psychology, 4*, 41–62.

Holmstom, C., Johnson, K., Dillion, J., Finch, J., Hothersall, S., Joseph, M., Meleyal, L., Neville, R., Wiles, F. (2014). Assessing the suitability of students to enter and remain on qualifying social work programmes: Guidance for universities and their employer partners in England. The Higher Education Academy, The Joint University Vouncil Social Work Education Committee and the College of Social Work.

Jameson, J. (2012). Leadership values, trust and negative capability: Managing the uncertainties of future English higher education. *Higher Education Quarterly, 66,* 391–414.

Keashly, L., & Neuman, J. H. (2010). Faculty experiences with bullying in higher education. *Administrative Theory & Praxis, 32,* 48–70.

Khoo, S. (2010). Academic mobbing: Hidden health hazard at the workplace. *Malaysian Family Physician: The Official Journal of the Academy of Family Physicians of Malaysia, 5,* 61–67.

Levidow, L. (2002). Marketizing higher education: Neoliberal strategies and counter-strategies. In K. Robins & F. Webster (Eds.), *The virtual university? Knowledge, markets, and management* (pp. 227–248). Oxford: Oxford University Press.

Luttrell, W. (2005). Crossing anxious borders: Teaching across the quantitative-qualitative "divide". *International Journal of Research & Method in Education, 28,* 183–195.

Parker, I. (1998). Realism, relativism and critique in psychology. In I. Parker (Ed.), *Social constructionism, discourse and realism* (pp. 1–10). London: SAGE Publications.

Parker, I. (2013). Discourse analysis: Dimensions of critique in psychology. *Qualitative Research in Psychology, 10,* 223–239.

Parker, I. (2014). *Discourse dynamics: Critical analysis for social and individual psychology.* London: Routledge.

Perlin, M. L. (2006). International human rights law and comparative mental disability law: The universal factors. *Syracuse Journal of International Law and Commerce, 34,* 333.

Phillips, J. C., & Fischer, A. R. (1998). Graduate students' training experiences with lesbian, gay, and bisexual issues. *The Counseling Psychologist, 26,* 712–734.

Phoenix, A. (1994). Practicing feminist research: The intersection of gender and "race" in the research process. In M. Maynard & J. Purvis (Eds.), *Researching women's lives from a feminist perspective* (pp. 49–71). London: Taylor & Francis.

Pilgrim, D. (2007). The survival of psychiatric diagnosis. *Social Science & Medicine, 65,* 536–547.

Poole, J. M., Jivraj, T., Arslanian, A., Bellows, K., Chiasson, S., Hakimy, H., et al. (2012). Sanism, mental health, and social work/education: A review and call to action. *Intersectionalities: A Global Journal of Social Work Analysis, Research, Polity, and Practice, 1,* 20–36.

Povee, K., & Roberts, L. D. (2014). Qualitative research in psychology: Attitudes of psychology students and academic staff. *Australian Journal of Psychology, 66,* 28–37.

Quality Assurance Agency for Higher Education (2010). *Subject benchmark statement: Psychology.* Gloucester: Author.

Reid, J., & Poole, J. (2013). Mad students in the social work classroom? Notes from the beginnings of an inquiry. *Journal of Progressive Human Services, 24,* 209–222.

Rose, N. (1979). The psychological complex: Mental measurement and social administration. *Ideology & Consciousness, 5,* 5–68.

Sedivy-Benton, A., Strohschen, G., Cavazos, N., & Boden-Mcgill, C. (2015). Good ol' boys, mean girls, and tyrants. *Adult Learning, 26,* 35–41.

Shaw, R., Dyson, P., & Peel, E. (2008). Qualitative psychology at M level: A dialogue between learner and teacher. *Qualitative Research in Psychology, 5*, 179–191.

Sin, C. H., & Fong, J. (2009). The impact of regulatory fitness requirements on disabled social work students. *British Journal of Social Work, 39*, 1518–1539.

Smith, D. (1986). Institutional ethnography: A feminist method. *Resources for Feminist Research, 15*, 6–13.

Smith, D. (2005). *Institutional ethnography: A sociology for people*. New York: Altamira.

Spandler, H., & Anderson, J. (2015). Unreasonable adjustments? Applying disability policy to madness and distress. In H. Spandler, J. Anderson, & B. Sapey (Eds.), *Madness, distress and the politics of disablement* (pp. 13–26). Bristol: University of Bristol Press.

Symons, S. (2013). Discursive constructions of UK swingers' self-identities and practices in a culturally gendered mononormative context. *Psychology of Women Section Review, 15*, 40–46.

Thornicroft, G. (2006). *Shunned: Discrimination against people with mental illness*. Oxford: Oxford University Press.

Tosh, J. (2011). The medicalization of rape: A discursive analysis of "paraphilic coercive disorder" and the psychiatrization of sexuality. *Psychology of Women Section Review, 13*, 2–12.

Tosh, J. (2013). The (in)visibility of childhood sexual abuse: Psychiatric theorizing of transgenderism and intersexuality. *Intersectionalities: A Global Journal of Social Work Analysis, Research, Polity, and Practice, 2*, 71–87.

Tosh, J. (2015). *Perverse psychology: The pathologization of sexual violence and transgenderism*. London: Routledge.

Tosh, J. (2016). *Psychology and gender dysphoria: Feminist and transgender perspectives*. London: Routledge.

Tosh, J., Brodie, A., Small, E., & Sprigings, K. (2014). "Why did I spend years learning all that rubbish, when I could have been doing this?" Student experiences of discourse analysis and feminist research. *Psychology of Women Section Review, 16*, 6–8.

Voss, J., & Gannon, L. (1978). Sexism in the theory and practice of clinical psychology. *Professional Psychology, 9*, 623–632.

Webb, S. A. (2006). *Social work in a risk society: Social and political perspectives*. New York: Palgrave Macmillan.

Weedon, C. (1996). *Feminist practice and poststructuralist theory*. London: Wiley.

CHAPTER 9

Creating the Better Workplace in Our Minds: Workplace "Mental Health" and the Reframing of Social Problems as Psychiatric Issues

Rob Wipond and Sonya Jakubec

INTRODUCTION

It has become commonplace in North America to portray worker "mental health" as one of the most significant problems facing workers, employers, and the economy. The Canadian Institutes of Health Research (2007) reports that there is "a looming crisis in health care and worker productivity that will result in severe economic consequences" (p. 5). "Mental health" and "alcohol abuse disorders," they write, "are the sleeping giant of health care in modern society" that "will create immense problems for the individuals with these conditions and for the companies who employ them" (p. 1). The Mental Health Commission of Canada states:

> The total cost from mental health problems and illnesses to the Canadian economy is conservatively estimated to be at least $50 billion per year. This represents 2.8 % of GDP. ... [C]umulative costs over the next 30 years are expected to exceed $2.3 trillion in current dollars. ... About 21.4 % of the working population currently experience mental health problems and illnesses that potentially affect their work productivity. ... A conservative estimate of the impact of mental health problems and illnesses on lost productivity due to absenteeism, presenteeism (present but less than fully productive at work) and turnover [was] about $6.3B in 2011 ... this will

R. Wipond (✉)
Victoria, BC, Canada
e-mail: rob@robwipond.com

S. Jakubec
School of Nursing and Midwifery, Mount Royal University, Calgary, AB, Canada

© The Editor(s) (if applicable) and The Author(s) 2016   161
B. Burstow (ed.), *Psychiatry Interrogated*,
DOI 10.1007/978-3-319-41174-3_9

rise to $16B in 2041. ... Mental health problems and illnesses typically account for approximately 30 % of short- and long-term disability claims. (2013a, p. XX)

Such pointedly ominous assertions are part of growing national and international discussions that are becoming increasingly visible in academic literature, advertising, news media, business conferences, public education efforts, and workplaces themselves.

Over the past two decades there has been a flurry of studies related to workplace mental health internationally; for instance, in Australia (Shann et al. 2014), the United Kingdom (Paton 2009), Canada (Dimoff and Kelloway 2013), the United States (Greenberg et al. 2015), and in relation to non-Western global contexts (Chopra 2009). There has been a recent proliferation of research, action guides, and working papers on workplace "mental health" in Canada in particular (Mental Health Commission of Canada 2012; Great West Life Centre for Mental Health in the Workplace 2013). Conferences, such as the Conference Board of Canada's "The Better Workplace," the Mental Health Commission of Canada's 2014 webinar series, and a cross-country panel (Economic Club of Canada 2015), are all examples of the upsurge of calls for action on "mental health" in workplace settings.

Many of the core ideas have become culturally commonplace and are aptly summarized in a promotional video for the Chokka Center for Integrative Health (Chokka 2014). The speaker in the video states: "On any given week, more than 500,000 Canadians will not go to work because of poor mental health." Double that number, the speaker adds, will be suffering "presenteeism." Associated stigma, delays in getting treatment, lack of supports, lack of insurance parity with respect to physical injuries, and loss of productivity, the speaker explains, all add up to the fact that "mental health issues are the single largest challenge facing employers today." These realities, the speaker argues, present both a serious threat to the bottom line and, conversely, a promise of significant financial returns for the savvy investor:

> Effective treatments for these conditions exist. Treatments which are scientifically proven to work, and that result in as much as a 270 % return on your investment for every dollar your company spends on prevention (Chokka 2014, n.p.).

An unequivocally positive "business case" is often presented by others in similar ways, including the Mental Health Commission of Canada, Canadian Standards Association, and the Bureau de Normalisation du Quebec (2013):

> Employees will clearly benefit from workplaces that promote and protect their psychological health and safety. For employers, the business case rests on four main parameters—enhanced cost effectiveness, improved risk management, increased organizational recruitment and retention as well as corporate social responsibility. (pp. 1–2)

Such incitements are more than just strong rhetorical encouragements—they frequently develop into demonstrable legal, financial, and political pressures on people to take action to prevent negative repercussions. For example, insurance organizations that manage employee services have put increased pressure on employers, who in turn have pressured medical practitioners (Baker 2014).

Shain (2010) cites influential precedents such as an Ontario court ruling in favor of an employee who, upon disclosing to his employer that he had "bipolar disorder," was terminated, and then plunged into a "manic episode" and was hospitalized. Shain further points to a British Columbia Workers Compensation Appeals Tribunal that ordered a court review of policies with respect to compensation for "chronic mental injury" (2010, p. XX). A Mental Health Commission of Canada (MHCC) action guide (2012) for employers lists some of the alleged consequences of failing to take action with regard to workplace mental health:

> ... possible loss of skilled employees; regulatory or legal sanctions for failing to recognize and make reasonable efforts to avert work-related injuries or incidents; escalating costs related to increased benefits utilization, lost productivity, recruitment and replacement expenses, and insurance premiums; negative impact on employee morale and engagement, customer and client relations, and organizational reputation. (p. 2)

In summary, North American workplace "mental health" exhortations are becoming rife with attention-grabbing, almost-utopian promises for curative impacts. The exhortations also are being couched in threats and fears that paint almost catastrophic potential consequences from inaction.

These are not unfamiliar refrains to anyone knowledgeable about North America's dominant mental health system. In addition, they hint at a disjuncture. Previous explorations of "mental health" discourse (Jakubec 2004; Jakubec and Campbell 2003; Jakubec and Rankin 2014) and "mental health" policy and practice (Wipond 2012, 2013a,b, 2014a,b,c, 2015) flagged many potential concerns about what workplace "mental health" initiatives have actually been inducing in the real world beyond such rhetoric. We knew, for example, that the dominant Western mental health system is itself a deeply contested space characterized by polarized power relationships between the providers and the people actually receiving the "treatments" or services. In addition, profound political tensions are built into federal, provincial, and state laws that allow assertive, coercive, and forced "mental health care."

Furthermore, extremely divergent opinions and struggles for power emerge in the scientifically unvalidated diagnostic methods and the often unreliable, ineffective, and demonstrably dangerous treatment practices (Wipond 2013b; Breggin 2008; Summerfield 2008). So, we asked, could importing principles, policies, and practices from the mental health system into workplaces truly, as suggested, "create and continually improve a psychologically healthy and safe workplace?" (Canadian Standards Association, 2013). Or were there in fact serious, inadequately discussed risks to implementing workplace "mental health" initiatives? Although we, as the researchers for this chapter, did not begin our investigation with the traditional institutional ethnography (IE) disjuncture discussed in Chapter 1, we very much had a sense of a disjuncture—and herein lay the conundrums that compelled us to investigate further.

METHODS

The study began informally through observing colleagues and friends who were finding themselves in contentious workplace situations. We saw them struggling with increasing demands on their time, mounting responsibilities, uncertain contracts, conflicts with coworkers or managers, and other types of workplace challenges. Yet, for many of them, psychiatric evaluations and "treatments" became the only "solutions" that emerged. This prompted us to review the dominant literature and "boss texts" related to "workplace mental health" initiatives in Canada. We wanted to see whether or how they grappled with the challenges of distinguishing between actual, legitimate problems located in workplaces, and problems allegedly located only in the "unhealthy minds" of workers.

The study then formally began when the second author participated in "The Better Workplace" conference in Calgary, Alberta (Conference Board of Canada 2015), the Conference Board of Canada's 18th annual gathering focused on "wellness, change and corporate culture." This conference provided an overview of the main ways in which workplace mental health initiatives were being discussed, along with many links to institutions, prominent people in the field, and influential reference documents. Informed by this conference, data for this study include several publicly available boss documents and three expert informant interviews conducted in May and June of 2015.

Text Analysis: Impact of a "Mental Health" Continuum that Lacks Points of Clarity

As alluded to earlier, our literature review highlighted the growing interest in workplace "mental health" internationally (LaMontagne et al. 2014) and in Canada (Dimoff and Kelloway 2013; Human Resources and Skills Development Canada 2011). We found that concepts of worker productivity (Paton 2009) and absenteeism and presenteeism (Schultz and Edington 2007) commonly stand out. Individual and workplace interventions based on managing "mental illness" (McDowell and Fossey 2015) and promoting broader "mental health" and wellness (LaMontagne et al. 2014) predominate. In particular, the *continuum model*, addressing a spectrum of health and illness issues (Jovanović 2015; Keyes 2002, 2007), has been given a largely unquestioned centrality in the evolving workplace mental health discourse.

The continuum model outlines a spectrum of mental conditions from "psychological health" to "mental illness." The model identifies points along the spectrum as to when, where, and which type of action is required to maximize psychological well-being. According to Lamers (2012), the continuum model has roots in several common "mental health" tools used to assess emotional, psychological, and social well-being in the general population. The model also has roots in the mental health system's expanding diagnostic categories, or in what some call a trend toward "diagnostic inflation" that allows increasing numbers of "ordinary" people to be labeled as having "mental disorders" (Kudlow 2013). The model also reflects the system's growing emphasis on early identification and intervention for "premorbid" conditions—that is, well before people have developed any diagnosed "mental illness" (Andreasen et al. 1992; Chwastiak et al. 2010, 2011).

In our text analyses, we identified a series of related Canadian texts in which the mental health continuum model consistently plays a central role. The version of the model that is integrated into these documents, along with an associated diagram, originated from the Canadian Armed Forces (CAF). The National Defence and the Canadian Armed Forces (NDCAF) site (2013) uses colors to explain the mental health spectrum:

> Recent experiences have taught us that many CAF members have physical and mental health concerns that, if identified and treated early, have the potential to be temporary and reversible. This model recognizes the spectrum of health concerns ... from health, adaptive coping (green), through mild and reversible distress or functional impairment (yellow), to more severe, persistent injury or impairment (orange), to clinical illnesses and disorders requiring more concentrated medical care (red) (p. XX).

The diagram includes arrows pointing in both directions along the spectrum from green through yellow and orange to red, emphasizing that people can move back and forth between "health" and "clinical illnesses." Accompanying text emphasizes that interventions occur as people slide toward "clinical mental illness" or the red zone, and that the earlier such interventions occur, "the easier" it is for people "to return to full health and functioning," as represented by the green zone (NDCAF 2013).

Several key documents developed in partnership with the Mental Health Commission of Canada (MHCC) incorporate this specific "mental health continuum" model. These documents have been widely distributed for use in Canadian workplaces (see Figure 9.1). The highest level text is "Psychological health and safety in the workplace—Prevention, promotion, and guidance to staged implementation," referred to by the MHCC as "the Standard" (Canadian Standards Association 2013). Developed through a process involving various stakeholders and in collaboration with the Canadian Standards Association, according to the MHCC it is the first nationally sanctioned voluntary standard that provides a set of principles for workplace mental health and safety. The document, "Assembling the Pieces—An Implementation Guide to the National Standard for Psychological Health and Safety in the Workplace"

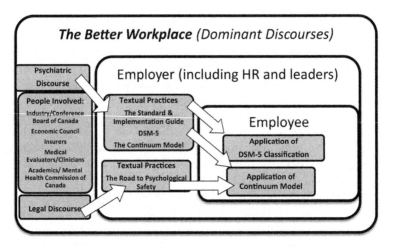

Figure 9.1   The social organization of workplace "mental health" initiatives in Canada

(Canadian Standards Association 2014), is a follow-up text to the "Standard," and it provides a set of general implementation guidelines for employers.

The Standard defines "mental health" and "psychological health" as "a state of well-being in which the individual realizes his or her own abilities, can cope with the normal stresses of life, can work productively and fruitfully, and is able to make a contribution to his or her community" (p. 4). Alongside that, psychological safety is "the absence of harm and/or threat of harm to mental well-being that a worker might experience" (Canadian Standards Association 2014, p. 4).

The vague, normative, and value-laden aspects of terms (e.g., "abilities," "cope," "productively," "normal," and "harm to mental well-being") pass without critical analysis, leaving an infinite trail of questions in their wake. For example, if "harm" to some people's "mental well-being" can be caused by someone pointing to disturbing facts, does that mean that workplace environments should minimize dealing with hard facts? Do working "productively" by social measures and working truly "fruitfully" by personal measures sometimes exist at cross-purposes? Is it "normal" and "healthy" to feel a state of "well-being" while performing a job that contributes environmental pollution into one's community? Are minimum-wage pay and constant threats of greater impoverishment "normal" stressors that workers *should be able to comfortably* accept and cope with, or should workers regard them as intolerable and unacceptable?

The lack of any attempts to grapple with such questions is a convincing indication that the "Standard" and "Implementation Guide" are not designed to help employers and employees critically and democratically develop their own creative, innovative approaches toward increasing mutual psychological self-understanding. Instead, the texts seem to mainly serve as encouragements for employers and employees to import dominant standards about productivity, normality, psychological harm, and "mental health" from the broader society and the "mental health" system deeper into the workplace.

Now, words like *mental illness* are not in the dominant vocabulary—in fact they are largely purged and/or disclaimed. Still, strange though it may seem to say this, the purging from all of the texts of any attempts to grapple with what "*mental illness*" is, even while the concept is central to the entire effort, itself constitutes further evidence that the texts serve primarily as conduits for the importing of normative "mental health" system standards. For example, the term "*mental illness*" per se is neither in the glossary nor prevalent in these two boss texts. Instead, the phrases "psychological well-being," "psychological health and safety," and sometimes "mental health" dominate. According to the Implementation Guide of the Canadian Standards Association (2014):

> Is this about worker mental illness? No. Adopting a PHSMS [Psychological Health and Safety Management System] isn't about assessing a worker's mental health. It is about considering the impact of workplace processes, policies, and interactions on the psychological health and safety of all workers. For those workers who have a mental illness such as depression or anxiety, there may be other things for an employer to consider, like the duty to accommodate described in human rights legislation. ... Although a PHSMS can be helpful for workers with mental illness, a PHSMS is primarily intended to be preventive for the entire workforce in the same way that occupational health and safety systems are preventive for physical injuries and illnesses for the entire workforce. (p. XX)

What we are suggesting is that the purging of the term "mental illness" is deliberate on the surface so that these two texts can seem more relevant, inviting, and applicable to all workers wherever they are on the "mental health" continuum.

It is likewise relevant that this superficial purging is not fundamental to the MHCC workplace "mental health" effort as a whole. For example, by contrast, there are a variety of research backgrounders, brochures, promotional leaflets, and other MHCC-distributed documents that serve to introduce, advertise, or supplement the two boss texts, and many of these explain that the "Standard" and "Implementation Guide" indeed are intended to aid in the prevention and management of "mental illnesses."

In "The Road to Psychological Safety," a MHCC research backgrounder, the authors contend that the perfect workplace would have both a broader psychological wellness strategy and a strategy for dealing with "mental illness" (Mental Health Commission of Canada 2013b). An associated resource, "Psychological Health and Safety: An Action Guide for Employers," is specifically concerned with methods for supporting and managing employees who have been diagnosed with "mental disorders."

Despite these superficial differences, what is consistent throughout all of the texts is that there is a clearly articulated spectrum passing from health to "illness," with a complete lack of rigorous explication or critical analyses of the meanings of these very terms. Besides, the authors of these texts consistently sidestep key questions that their own "mental health" continuum model inevitably raises. Namely, if people can move back and forth along the entire continuum, then for practical purposes in actual circumstances it is vital to understand when a person is crossing from one point on the spectrum to the other, and who will determine that and how. To put this simply, when is something a "normal response" to harm or adversity? When is it "mental illness"? And who decides? More specifically, which criteria does one use to distinguish between (1) a person who is struggling with reasonable levels of anxiety or depression as a result of genuine, unreasonably demanding challenges or conflicts in the workplace; (2) a person who is suffering from the "mental disorders" of anxiety and depression, and is only looking for reasonable accommodation; and (3) a person who is suffering but is nonetheless demanding too much accommodation?

To us, the fact that such clearly relevant issues and tensions are unexplored in the MHCC texts, while key terms and models from the mental health system enter unquestioned into the boss texts, suggested that the "Standard" and "Implementation Guide" serve mainly as conduits for importing dominant "mental health" system diagnostic and treatment standards into workplaces. We suspected, therefore, that initiatives using these or similar approaches would simultaneously also import many of the profound problems and conflicts of the dominant mental health system into workplaces. In addition, as we soon saw, our expert informants strongly affirmed that this is exactly what is happening in the field.

From Texts to the Everyday World: What Effects Do "Mental Health" Initiatives Actually Have in Workplaces?

The dominance of the "mental health continuum model" in the texts, alongside poorly defined terms of psychological health and illness, suggested to us that the same concepts and tensions inherent in the dominant mental health system had the potential to be "imported" into workplace "mental health" initiatives. So then, what sort of problems, if any, would this actually lead to in everyday settings? As evidenced in the texts, and as we knew to be typical of the mental health system, we suspected that we would see at least three key impacts in workplace settings from the use of approaches drawn from the dominant "mental health" system:

- Evidence of *coercion*, of employees being invited into dialogues about "psychological well-being" that were in fact little more than thinly masked attempts to draw them into processes of labeling and self-labeling with "mental disorders" or "early signs" of "mental disorders"
- People *reframing* workplace social conflicts as symptoms of personal "mental disorders," much like the dominant mental health system reframes the impacts on individuals of trauma, poverty, or other problematic social circumstances as "disorders" arising from "chemical imbalances"

- Increased use of "mental health" *diagnostic labels* and, alongside that, increases in discriminatory behaviors reflective of common prejudices in broader society about people with "mental disorders"

INTERVIEW DATA AND ANALYSIS

We interviewed Brian, Christine, and Debbie (all pseudonyms). These three would be considered to be "workplace mental health" experts. Brian was trained as a counsellor and therapist, and later became a consultant to organizations and businesses on "mental health" disability claims. At the time of the interview he was a senior executive at an independent medical exam company often hired by employers to intervene in disability and mental health-related cases. Christine was a human resources professional with 20 years of experience working with a variety of organizations and firms, with the number of employees ranging from 100 to more than 10,000. She participated in "mental health" and wellness-related education and training, along with workplace disability management (e.g., accommodations and terminations). Trained in education and counseling, Debbie became a wellness specialist at a large Canadian corporation. At the time of the interview she was a "mental health" coordinator at a large university. She also served in advisory roles to several other leading national mental health organizations concerned with education and policy development.

Inviting Separation of "Psychological Well-Being" from "Mental Illness"

As previously described, some parts of the Mental Health Commission of Canada's texts seem to create a sharp divide between dealing with challenges to "mental well-being" or "psychological wellness" in the workplace on the one hand, and dealing with "clinical mental illness" on the other. Other parts of MHCC texts place these concepts on a continuum and indicate that people can readily move from one extreme to the other in both directions. At no point do the texts explicitly grapple with this apparent contradiction or with the philosophical, sociological, and scientific challenges of accurately defining or understanding any of these concepts. We wanted to know how and why people working in the field handled these concepts—as distinctly divided, or as existing on a continuum—and what the effects were of handling the terms the way that they did.

Brian and Christine were unaware of the specific MHCC documents and indicated that they and their professional associates mostly used the primary texts of their respective professions. For example, Brian described his company's "mental health" professionals using common psychiatric diagnostic tests and the company's legal professionals using texts related to disability law. This was important, because we knew that common psychiatric diagnostic tests placed "mental health" and "mental illness" on a continuum, and the dividing line was simply an arbitrary cut-off score between ill and well. The increasingly common psychiatric use of terms, such as "mild depression" or "moderate mental illness," further blurred the lines along the continuum. Nevertheless, notably, like some of the higher-level MHCC documents do, both Brian and Christine explained that they often employed a sharper conceptual division between "psychological wellness" and "mental illness," and Debbie elaborated on this particularly clearly.

Debbie was the only interviewee who identified using specific workplace "mental health" documents in her work—the MHCC's "The Working Mind" (Mental Health Commission of Canada 2015). She was also an advisor to the MHCC, and described some of the thinking behind how the MHCC handled the concepts of "psychological health" and "mental illness" in a different way. "Mental illness," she stated, is generally perceived to be something bearing considerable stigma, while affecting only a small minority. This has proven to be not only a roadblock in promoting discussions about mental illness in the workplace, explained Debbie, but has even raised the spectre that such discussions may be backfiring by increasing anxiety and stereotyped labeling among workers.

Debbie explained that the MHCC has been studying whether programs like theirs, which emphasize terms and concepts associated with "mental illnesses," are helping. She stated:

> They are actually starting to look at the data from these courses [such as Mental Health First Aid] and they're starting to ask, 'Does this course actually increase stigma?' (Interview, April 2015).

Consequently, she explained: "'The Working Mind' program does put 'mental illness' at one end of a continuum opposite mental wellness; however, the program emphasizes the concepts and language of maintaining 'psychological health' and well-being because these terms seem to be more universal and culturally acceptable." In the interview, Debbie went on to say:

> We're no longer offering *mental health* per se. It just wasn't meeting the needs of the participants. But "The Working Mind" is what we are focusing on. ... It's actually designed for employees, and it's a three-and-a-half hour program that really looks at health on a continuum. It gives indicators as to what goes on for ourselves when we are not well. What does that look like? What does that feel like? ... And then [employees] have a common language like, "Oh, I think I am in the yellow zone today," or "I'm moving into the orange zone," and each of these zones represents a different sort of place of well-being. ... There's a way that it's presented, the language that's used, it puts people at ease. It takes a lot for someone to say, "You know I've been having a lot of anxiety." They might not feel comfortable saying that, but what you do hear is things like, "I haven't been sleeping." ... And then we can have a discussion about that and talk about sleep hygiene and how sleep affects us and things like that. I think it is really about providing more of a common language that people are comfortable in using.

In effect, she explained, "The Working Mind" was a program about preventing and dealing with "mental illnesses," *framed* as a program about maintaining psychological well-being because conversations about psychological health were seen to be less stigmatizing, less stigmatized, and more "normal," and therefore more likely to be readily accepted in workplace environments. Notably, Brian and Christine regarded it similarly but without even being aware of the Mental Health Commission texts. Brian said:

> It's okay to tell your colleagues that you had a brush with cancer, but mentioning a brush with mental health issues, depression, anxiety—which are two of the most common types of issues in the workplace for employees—it's not as easy to fess up to. (Interview, May 2015)

So one goal of his work, said Brian, was to help make practices that promote "psychological health"—as preventative of "mental illnesses"—become normalized and recognized as part of everyone's daily routine. According to Brian, in the same interview, this goal involved:

> ...[H]elping employers and employees get to a place where mental health, where conversations around mental health, become like any other [occupational] safety meeting in the morning. ... (T)he more we can normalize those conversations, the stronger individuals and employers will be to work together as employees do go through some kind of mental health crises.

In this way, irrespective of the degree of awareness involved, "workplace mental health" programs were being presented as concerned with "psychological well-being," mainly as a way to more effectively invite, coerce, or seduce people into discussions of issues pertaining to early identification and treatment of "mental illnesses."

Workplace Mental Health Initiatives Often Involve Coercion and Pressure

Some of the workplace "mental health" educational and training programs discussed with the interviewees were simply made available to workers, which was why an "inviting" language and framing was important. Yet, these programs were hardly voluntary, for they were firmly embedded within the existing power dynamics of the organizations that implemented them. Debbie explained that, usually, such programs would be mandated into existence by senior directors at large organizations, and then employees were often "asked" or directed to participate in the programs by their managers.

Additional pressures could emerge, she explained, because alleged financial drains caused by "mental health" problems were a primary argument used to persuade employers to launch such initiatives; consequently, organizations wanted to see financial returns on their investments. This then led directly to expanding expectations, coercion, and pressure on employees to be "mentally well" at all times, especially once they had received supposedly effective training.

This kind of pressure compounded her own anxieties and self-criticism and ultimately contributed to Debbie having a personal psychological crisis herself at one point. She described her personal experience during the interview in this way:

> I was quite sick and ended up being hospitalized, and all of that. … It was difficult because it felt like I should know what to do and take care of myself to prevent this from happening.

So coercion, pressure of expectation, and force have become key parts of workplace mental health initiatives, in a similar way to how coercion, pressure, and force are key parts of the dominant "mental health" system.

Reframing Workplace Difficulties and Conflicts as "Mental Health" Problems

Many of the texts we examined portray "mental health" approaches as helping resolve many types of difficulties and conflicts in the workplace (i.e., if employees start feeling more psychologically healthy, they will have fewer problems at work). Nevertheless, workplace institutional structures in an oligarchical capitalist society tend to be strong and resistant to change. Therefore, in light of the blurred lines about what "mental illness" or "mental health" even are, it seemed to us equally, if not more likely, that focusing on individuals' "mental health" in conflict situations would become a way to divert attention and energy away from relatively intransigent political, economic, and structural issues of the workplace. It could, we surmised, draw more intense attention toward individuals' internal experiences, struggles, and self-blaming. Our interviews proved that to be the case.

Brian did describe instances of employees' psychological struggles leading to recommendations for accommodations. However, the interviewees more often, and much more powerfully, described situations where the influence went in the opposite direction. Employees' struggles with their own minds and experiences most often became focal, while senior leaders and the workplace environment that they controlled continued to resist change.

Christine, for example, said senior leaders were often "untouchable" during situations of workplace conflict; thus, the focus would turn to lower-level workers' increasing psychological distress and self-defined "mental health." This happened to Christine herself. In this regard she stated: "I was in a situation where I was being effectively bullied by a senior leader who was very connected and powerful within the organization." She could not even bring this senior manager into conflict-resolution discussions, and so started to suffer severe psychological distress. "I was having significant symptoms related to anxiety. I was not functioning in the workplace anymore. I was requiring medication to go from my car to my office in the morning. I was having panic attacks. I was having severe insomnia," Christine said.

As soon as she quit working at the company, though, Christine said she experienced a deep, enduring feeling of release from the distress: "The issue wasn't that I was mentally ill ... the issue was that I worked in a horrible environment that raised my stress to an unmanageable level." Similarly, Debbie's own latent, personal "mental health" problems, she said, blossomed into serious "mental illness" for a period of time because of workplace conditions that she felt she could not change. She explained:

> I think it has to do with pressure and performance. You add on the extra stress of this job which was quite a lot of responsibility. I really enjoyed it, but the added pressure and then working kind of in isolation. I didn't have a team here. ... Our team was all spread out. It felt like you were paddling your own canoe. That was not good for me.

The increasing tendency of employers to turn to "mental health" approaches as a way to try to defuse or diminish the impact of institutional pressures and conflicts was often thinly veiled. Debbie explained that her current employer funded a major workplace mental health initiative at the same time as senior leaders began putting more responsibilities on employees. In concert with these changes she noticed more employees turning to her for help and having apparent "mental health" problems emerge amid the increasing stress and anxiety. According to Debbie:

> There's a lot of pressure on [employees], and there have been a lot of changes. Some [employees] are, well, it was put to me, they're crushed. They're so demoralized.

The use of "mental health" approaches to manage collective employee reactions to potentially harmful institutional decisions was particularly evident in a situation in which Brian was involved. A large organization was about to announce a significant "downsizing" that included firing many employees. Brian was hired to meet with the organization's human resources team and coach them on how to deliver the announcements to key employees at group meetings. He then facilitated those meetings and led ensuing group discussions among the employees, helping people deal with their "emotional reactions." Brian's description was telling as he emphasized his role in redirecting the workers' attention:

> I was there to facilitate, along with the employer, sessions with these employees and put out the facts, get the individuals' personal reaction to it. Keep it away from the operational side, focusing (instead) on the individual's personal reaction to that and helping the individuals move through that. ... Just really helping the individual go through that process. ... We were running these every 90 minutes [each] day, so six or seven sessions. ... It helps people go from a place of facts, personal reactions, and then go down into the emotional side of it, and then help build people back up to, "So how do we leave this room and how do we move forward?"

Brian said the feedback from the employer later was that employees found it to be a "very respectful process" in which they felt "heard and understood," while they also reportedly came to a better understanding of the challenges the employer was facing.

Mass firings can often trigger deep frustrations and anxieties in workers, and incite shared discussions that may lead, for example, to collective protests about power inequities, accusations against managers, or calls for change to fundamental aspects of company financial decision making. This is precisely what such "mental health" reframings effectively prevent. Brian's role was to carefully coach the employees into regarding the financial situation of the company and the downsizing decisions as immutable "facts" and to focus their reactions instead on changing and moving past their immediate "individual" feelings. The extent to which the tactics "worked" for many remaining or fired employees could be regarded as a measure of many workers' growing acceptance of turning to such individualized psychotherapeutic approaches in the face of social challenges.

Workplace Mental Health Initiatives Can Lead to Increases in Diagnosed "Mental Disorders," Disability Claims, and Summary Firings

The main texts that we reviewed instruct employers and employees in words and concepts that emphasize particular ways of viewing workplace difficulties and conflicts. The boss documents frame workplace challenges as if they are being created and perpetuated by minds that are not sufficiently "psychologically healthy," are not supporting "psychological health" enough, or are in fact "mentally disordered." Then, what are the repercussions of this in the field?

We found that categorizing workplace problems as "mental health" problems automatically recontextualized them in several other ways as well. All three interviewees highlighted the far-reaching impacts of these recontextualizations under the law. Essentially, identifying problems as "biochemical/physical" and "medical" made them subject to laws governing privacy, disability, and discrimination, which in turn led to further repercussions.

First, as soon as an employee's workplace-related problem became subject to medical privacy laws, it became shrouded in secrecy and mysticism for the coworkers and employers; and consequently often it was not easy for them to even try to accommodate. Christine explained it this way:

> [W]hen I say groups like (third-party medical claim managers) are a curse, they are great tools when you're looking at giving people privacy and anonymity, but as a result there is complete privacy and anonymity ... so nobody actually knows what the issues are and what you are dealing with. So you never have the ability to equip a team or a leader to deal with or help someone cope with return to the workplace or just being in the workplace because of this shroud of secrecy around the whole topic.

Brian, who worked at such a third-party company, effectively confirmed the dynamic complexities and challenges that medical privacy laws often created in resolving mental health-related workplace situations.

Second, employees were more readily seeking a "mental illness" diagnosis as a way of dealing with workplace problems, precisely because legislators and many organizations had created legal protections and procedures for people with formally defined "disabilities." Conversely, there were no comparable options for resolving serious conflicts that struck to the heart of power imbalances and other structural aspects of workplaces—particularly those between senior leaders and lower-level employees. As such, employees were being "set up" to actively participate in their own "psychiatrization." Brian pointed out that:

> Quite often we have found that the issue is related to conflict in the workplace—an employee having a conflict with their manager or supervisor. And the way it gets dealt with is unfortunately through the medical system. Which is how the current systems are set up, which is to push people to medicalize issues which should be dealt with on a behavioral level.

Sometimes employees were actually eager to embrace such self-psychiatrization, suggested Brian. He pointed to examples of employees getting poor performance evaluations, and then taking a medical leave for "mental health" reasons rather than dealing with it. He stated:

> [O]ften conflict in the workplace is medicalized rather than being dealt with as a behavioral issue. ... It's their way of confronting it. I can't call my boss an asshole, or bully, or whatever; I can go off on medical leave and not deal with it. It's a passive-aggressive approach to dealing with it. And unfortunately organizations can set up policies and procedures that support that kind of process versus a more clear process of dispute resolution. ... We often do that because that's the only route that's provided.

In addition, Brian explained that the unscientific aspects of "mental health" diagnostics supported such approaches. He described how this occurs:

> It's easier to get a mental health disability claim because nobody is looking at your broken arm or leg; it's what you have to say. And since I am angry at the workplace, I can make a mental health claim because that's the easiest route to getting permission to be away from work, and still be paid for a period of time. I think it's that simplistic.

The prompt pathologizing and medicalizing of these problems seemed almost assured by the system that was in place, explained Brian; it identified medical psychiatric professionals as the go-to experts. The requirement for legal clarity for employers, insurers, and others created a pressure to identify a "medical" diagnosis from the *Diagnostic and Statistical Manual of Mental Disorders* (DSM); consequently, psychiatric professionals with their medical training were regarded as the authorities. Brian reported that all third-party interlocuters recognized psychiatrists as having the most appropriate expertise over other types of "mental health" professionals. According to Brian:

> In our business it would just be a psychiatrist first and foremost. They may refer to an occupational psychologist or someone who works in rehab or something like that, but that may come as a secondary referral. ... Our role is to get a really clear diagnosis.

This in turn has led to a third significant impact in the workplace, as all three interviewees explained. When employers were officially informed that an employee had a diagnosed "mental health" problem, the employer now could not fire the employee for any cause, however valid, that might be related to the employee's disorder, because that would then be discrimination based on "disability." The employer had a "duty to accommodate" the employee under disability law so long as that accommodation did not cost the employer "undue hardship."

Christine explained that, with the vast diversity of types of "mental disorders" along with the wide-ranging breadth and depth of behavioral symptomologies that they encompassed, senior leaders at large, deep-pocketed companies often felt that their duty to accommodate could too easily get stretched and expanded by problematic employees far beyond the bounds of what the leaders would consider reasonable. At the same time, the texts of these same workplace "mental health" education programs, and the dominant mental health discourse in the broader culture, were usually giving employers the message that "mental illnesses" were organic "brain disorders" that were chronic and required lifelong treatment and management.

In effect, then, the company's troublesome employee now represented to senior leaders a virtually unbounded, incurable, perpetual demand for accommodation by an already low-performing employee. So increasingly, companies were simply buying such employees out. This common employee-buyout practice was described by Christine, who had worked regularly in human resource departments for companies. She explained:

> What if that employee wasn't performing well and you had intended to release him from the organization? And now you're aware you're dealing with a mental health issue. Are you going to have to keep them forever? These are the questions that I would get from the management. "Does that mean we have to keep them forever?" It's really kind of ugly ... (A)s soon as they know about it they have a requirement to accommodate it. ... I've had a number of conversations where I would describe a situation in general terms to an [employer], and they would be like, "Get rid of them." And I have to turn that "Get rid of them" into a situation where that won't garner us a lawsuit. ... I know that sounds horribly ugly, and I'm embarrassed to be a part of that world, really, but that's the reality.

The process of a buyout was accomplished in a number of ways, according to Christine:

What typically happens is that there is a side bar negotiation. [We] agree that the current workplace is no longer the ideal situation for that person to make a suitable recovery and be at their healthiest and we severance them out. ... That is just a side deal that happens to basically pay to make that situation go away.

Christine explained that under Canadian law, employees could be fired without cause so long as a large enough severance payment was made based on legal precedents. In this way she reflected: "A lot of these organizations deem it's easier—because they assume that if a person has mental health issues that they will be a quote un-quote re-occurring problem—it's easier to write a cheque." Christine said she had never in her career seen an employee who had received an actual "mental health" diagnosis get successfully accommodated by an employer instead of "severanced out."

Indeed, when she could not resolve her own conflicts with a senior manager and began to suffer intense psychological distress from it, Christine said she knew from experience that it would be relatively easy for her to get a diagnosis and then promptly get a large severance offer from the employer. Christine said she and her doctor reviewed the diagnoses available in the DSM and together settled on diagnosing her with "situational anxiety." According to Christine, "the workplace was just so toxic that it was extremely unhealthy to be there. I knew that when I returned to work, I would get a severance package." And she did.

In her own case, Debbie identified more strongly as having all along had an underlying, recurring "mental disorder," and she said she will "always wonder" whether one time when she was let go by an employer that it was because of her revealing her "mental health" diagnosis. "It definitely crossed my mind, and [the employer] of course wouldn't say that that was the reason," said Debbie; "and they were very generous in the severance package."

For his part, Brian indicated that he had seen successful workplace accommodations of people who had been diagnosed with "mental disorders." Still, significantly, he noted that these had usually occurred when a "correct diagnosis" had in turn helped to properly identify and uproot the "etiology" of a person's problem in the workplace conditions themselves such as "toxic manager, conflict with peers, etc." (personal communication, August 2015).

DISCUSSION

In our review of the literature and Canadian texts, we found that the "mental health continuum model" plays a central role in framing workplace "mental health" initiatives. In light of our understanding of the mental health system, we believed that the continuum model, rather than creating an ideal "Better Workplace," carried the risk of allowing some of the immensely troubled social relations endemic in the dominant system to be imported into workplace settings. Through interviews with employees, leaders, and participants in workplace "mental health" initiatives, we identified more clearly what those risks are, and how they are manifesting in workplace settings.

First, the lack of clear, scientifically valid definitions of either "psychological health" on one end of the spectrum or "mental illness" on the other leave both concepts wide open to interpretation. The result is that common understandings of "mental health" from the dominant mental health system and broader culture tend to get imported uncritically into workplace initiatives. In addition, the vague terms can be appropriated for a variety of other possible purposes within the relationships of power that are characteristic of most workplaces in modern capitalist society.

Second, coercive pressures are emerging for all employees to participate in "mental health" initiatives, in light of the alleged costs of "mental illness" to companies and the apparent threat that people can at any time slide along the continuum to become "mentally ill." This occurs in the same way that coercion and force are fundamental aspects of "early intervention" and "maintenance treatment" efforts in the dominant mental health system.

Third, the continuum model diverts attention from genuine management or labor problems in the workplace, and reframes workplace conflicts as being located somewhere on the spectrum of the psychological problems of individuals. This occurs basically in the same way that modern psychiatric approaches tend to highlight the individual's brain as the locus of concern for change rather than the social environment.

Finally, the continuum model polarizes "psychological health" and "mental illness" as distinctly different states of being at opposite extremes from each other. In that sense, the continuum polarizes and stigmatizes what it is purportedly intended to depolarize and de-stigmatize and creates a resultant deeper insolubility in conflict-resolution practices in workplaces. This creates a practical worsening of discrimination against people diagnosed with "mental illnesses": summary firings instead of mutual adaptation and accommodation, albeit with healthy severance packages.

Far from creating "an ideal workplace" then, the incorporation of "mental health" approaches into workplaces is having very different effects. It is diverting discussion from genuine labor and management issues, and reframing them as being located mainly in the troubled minds of the people who feel the most victimized by challenges, conflicts, and inequities of power.

These findings have particular significance for any employers, employees, human resource managers, unions, or others who are seeking to improve working conditions. The findings demonstrate that greater critical awareness and more nuanced approaches are required to properly understand the true impacts of workplace "mental health" initiatives—which would seem overall to be worsening rather than improving working conditions and fairness.

Another provocative possibility that our findings pointed to is that greater orientation and awareness among employees and employers of "mental health" concepts may explain the upsurge in recent years of mental health-related employment leaves and claims, more than any actual general worsening of workers' psychological health. Insofar as this is the case, workplace "mental health" initiatives are creating the very problem they are purporting to solve—namely, increasing the numbers of employees who are allegedly "mentally ill" and increasing the financial costs to companies.

Also of interest is the fact that all of this can take place even with the full awareness of the participants. That is, all of our interviewees were able to see and describe these contradictory results being produced by employing workplace "mental health" initiatives, but nonetheless still found a logic and value in participating in them. This speaks to the compelling power of the institutionalized practices driving the agenda, likely generated in no small part by the influential, widely permeating reach of mainstream "mental health" ideas in our society, the financial clout and public relations efforts of the pharmaceutical industry, and the unequal economic relations in modern capitalist workplaces.

CONCLUDING REMARKS

Under the guise of promoting an idealistic future of universally "psychologically healthy" workplaces, the "mental health continuum model" acts as a conduit to import ideas and ways of acting from the dominant "mental health" system into workplace settings. The result is that conflicts born in inequitable institutional, economic, and power relations are reframed as problems existing mainly in the minds and brains of individuals. This serves not to empower and liberate people from the actual problems of the workplace and the conditions of their work and social lives. It rather helps to gloss over their actual concerns, further isolating them, and making people even more vulnerable to the problems imposed on them by the institutional practices of "The Better Workplace."

REFERENCES

Andreasen, N. C., Flaum, M., & Arndt, S. (1992). The comprehensive assessment of symptoms and history (CASH): An instrument for assessing diagnosis and psychopathology. *Archives of General Psychiatry, 49*(8), 615.

Baker, R. (2014). *Accommodating mental illness and addictions at work balancing safety, human rights, performance and best medical care.* The Bottom Line Conference. Retrieved from http://www.bottomlineconference.ca/wp-content/uploads/2014/03/AccommodatingMentalIllnessandAddictionsatWork.pdf

Breggin, P. (2008). *Toxic psychiatry: Why therapy, empathy, and love must replace the drugs, electroshock, and biochemical theories of the "new psychiatry"* (2nd ed.). New York: Springer.

Canadian Institutes of Health Research (CIHR) Committee of Partners on Mental Health in the Workplace. (2007). *Mental health in the labour force: Literature review and research gap analysis.* Ottawa: Author. Retrieved from http://www.mental-healthroundtable.ca/jul_07/WW%20GAP%20Report%20-May30_2007.pdf

Canadian Standards Association Group. (2013). *The national standard for psychological health and safety in the workplace (the Standard).* Retrieved from http://shop.csa.ca/en/canada/occupational-healthand-safety-management/cancsa-z1003-13bnq-9700-8032013/invt/z10032013/?utm_source=redirect&utm_medium=vanity&utm_content=folder&utm_campaign=z1003#Download

Canadian Standards Association Group. (2014). *Assembling the pieces—An implementation guide to the national standard for psychological health and safety in the workplace* (The Implementation Guide). Retrieved from http://shop.csa.ca/en/canada/occupational-health-and-safety-management/cancsa-z1003-13bnq-9700-8032013/invt/27037012014.

Chwastiak, L. A., Rosenheck, R. A., & Kazis, L. E. (2011). Association of psychiatric illness and obesity, physical inactivity, and smoking among a national sample of veterans. *Psychosomatics, 52*, 230–236.

Chwastiak, L. A., Rosenheck, R. A., Desia, R., & Kazis, L. E. (2010). Association of psychiatric illness and all-cause mortality in the National Department of Veterans Affairs Health Care System. *Psychosomatic Medicine, 72*, 817–822.

Chokka, P. (2014). *Mental health in the workplace*. Chokka Center for Integrative Health. Retrieved from https://www.youtube.com/watch?v=z9c50z_R8dw&feature=youtu.be

Chopra, P. (2009). Mental health and the workplace: Issues for developing countries. *International Journal of Mental Health Systems, 3*(1), 4–4.

Conference Board of Canada. (2015). *The better workplace conference*. Retrieved from http://www.conferenceboard.ca/conf/betterworkplace/default.aspx.

Dimoff, J. K., & Kelloway, E. K. (2013). Bridging the gap: Workplace mental health research in Canada. *Canadian Psychology, 54*(4), 203.

Economic Club of Canada. (2015). *WELLth management: Mental health at work challenge, Calgary*. Retrieved from http://economicclub.ca/events/display/wellth-management-calgary

Great West Life Centre for Mental Health in the Workplace. (2013). *Defining workplace mental health needs: Responding with tools and resources*. Retrieved from https://www.workplacestrategiesformentalhealth.com/pdf/M7198_Defining_workplace_mental_health_needs.pdf

Greenberg, P. E., Fournier, A., Sisitsky, T., et al. (2015). The economic burden of adults with major depressive disorder in the United States (2005 and 2010). *The Journal of Clinical Psychiatry, 76*, 2, 155. Retrieved from http://www.psychiatrist.com/jcp/article/Pages/2015/v76n02/v76n0204.aspx

Human Resources and Skills Development Canada (2011). *Mental health in Canadian workplaces: Investigating employer's best practices*. Ottawa: Author/Great Place to Work® Institute Canada.

Jakubec, S. L. (2004). The "world mental health" framework: Dominant discourses in mental health and international development. *Canadian Journal of Community Mental Health, 23*(2), 23–38.

Jakubec, S. L., & Campbell, M. (2003). Mental health research and cultural dominance: An analysis of the social construction of knowledge for international development. *Canadian Journal of Nursing Research, 35*(2), 74–88.

Jakubec, S. L., & Rankin, J. M. (2014). Knowing the right to mental health: The social organization of research for global health governance. *Journal of Health Diplomacy, 1*(2), 1–22 Retrieved from http://www.ghd-net.org/sites/default/files/jakubec_rankin.pdf.

Jovanović, V. (2015). Structural validity of the mental health continuum-short form: The bifactor model of emotional, social and psychological well-being. *Personality and Individual Differences, 75*, 154–159.

Keyes, C. L. M. (2002). The mental health continuum: From languishing to flourishing in life. *Journal of Health and Social Behavior, 43*(2), 207–222.

Keyes, C. L. M. (2007). Promoting and protecting mental health as flourishing: A complementary strategy for improving national mental health. *American Psychologist*, *62*(2), 95–108.

Kudlow, P. (2013). The perils of diagnostic inflation. *Canadian Medical Association Journal—Journal De l'Association Medicale Canadienne*, *185*(1), E25–E26.

Lamers, S. M. A. (2012). *Positive mental health: Measurement, relevance and implications.* Enschede: University of Twente.

LaMontagne, A. D., Martin, A., Page, K. M., et al. (2014). Workplace mental health: Developing an integrated intervention approach. *BMC Psychiatry, 14*(1), 131–131.

Mental Health Commission of Canada. (2012). *Psychological health and safety and action guide for employers.* Retrieved from http://www.mentalhealthcommission.ca/English/system/files/private/document/Workforce_Employers_Guide_ENG.pdf

Mental Health Commission of Canada. (2013a). *Why investing in mental health will contribute to Canada's economic prosperity and to the sustainability of our health care system.* Retrieved at http://www.mentalhealthcommission.ca/English/node/742

Mental Health Commission of Canada. (2013b). *The road to psychological safety: Legal, scientific and social foundations for a national standard for psychological safety in the workplace.* Retrieved from http://www.mentalhealthcommission.ca/English/node/486

Mental Health Commission of Canada. (2015). *Initiatives and projects: The working mind.* Retrieved from http://www.mentalhealthcommission.ca/English/initiatives-and-projects/working-mind

Mental Health Commission of Canada, Canadian Standards Association, and the Bureau de Normalisation du Quebec. (2013). *The National Standard of Canada: Psychological health and safety in the workplace—Prevention, promotion and guidance to staged implementation: Frequently asked questions.* Retrieved from http://shop.csa.ca/en/canada/occupational-health-and-safety-management/cancsa-z1003-13bnq-9700-8032013/invt/z10032013 https://www.mentalhealthcommission.ca/English/system/files/private/document/MHCC_Standard_FAQ_ENG-1.pdf

McDowell, C., & Fossey, E. (2015). Workplace accommodations for people with mental illness: A scoping review. *Journal of Occupational Rehabilitation, 25*(1), 197–206.

National Defence and the Canadian Armed Forces. (2013). *The Military Mental Health Continuum Model.* Retrieved from http://www.forces.gc.ca/en/caf-community-health-services-r2mr-deployment/mental-health-continuum-model.page

Paton, N. (2009). *Poor mental health reduces workplace productivity levels.* Sutton: Reed Business Information UK.

Schultz, A. B., & Edington, D. W. (2007). Employee health and presenteeism: A systematic review. *Journal of Occupational Rehabilitation, 17*(33), 547–579.

Shain, M. (2010). *Tracking the Perfect Legal Storm: Converging legal systems create mounting pressure to create the psychologically safe workplace.* Mental Health Commission of Canada. Retrieved from https://www.mentalhealthcommission.ca/English/system/files/private/Workforce_Tracking_the_Perfect_Legal_Storm_ENG_0.pdf

Shann, C., Martin, A., & Chester, A. (2014). Improving workplace mental health: A training needs analysis to inform beyondblue online resource for leaders. *Asia Pacific, 52*(3), 298–315.

Summerfield, D. (2008). How scientifically valid is the knowledge base of global mental health? *BMJ, 336*, 992–994.

Wipond, R. (2015, February 18). Are America's high rates of mental illness actually based on sham science? *AlterNet*. Retrieved from http://www.alternet.org/personal-health/are-americas-high-rates-mental-illness-actually-based-sham-science

Wipond, R. (2014a, October 23). Research suggests that psychiatric interventions like admission to a mental facility could increase suicide risk. *AlterNet*. Retrieved from http://www.alternet.org/personal-health/research-suggests-psychiatric-interventions-admission-mental-facility-could-increase

Wipond, R. (2014b, July 7). The proactive search for mental illnesses in children. *Mad in America*. Retrieved from http://www.madinamerica.com/2014/07/proactive-pursuit/

Wipond, R. (2014c, July 9). The algorithmic managing of "at-risk" children. *Mad in America*. Retrieved from http://www.madinamerica.com/2014/07/algorithmic-management/

Wipond, R. (2013a). An overabundance of caution. *Focus*. Retrieved from http://www.focusonline.ca/?q=node/648

Wipond, R. (2013b, June 2013). Global psychiatric war hits home. *Focus*. Retrieved from http://focusonline.ca/?q=node/558

Wipond, R. (2012, November 2012). The case for electroshocking Mia. *Focus*. Retrieved from http://www.focusonline.ca/?q=node/463

Lawyering for the "Mad": Social Organization and Legal Representation for Involuntary-Admission Cases in Poland

Agnieszka Doll

In an interview with this author, a lawyer pointedly remarked that no one takes these legal aid cases willingly "because they require a lot of time, and the remuneration ... is simply laughable" (interview with attorney, January 22, 2013). Behind this comment is a very worrisome reality—namely, that Polish attorneys[1] experience legal aid lawyering in involuntary-admission cases as a burdensome and unproductive undertaking—all of which inevitably impacts negatively on the clients themselves. Attorneys commonly share the perception that remuneration is inadequate given the degree and quality of service required. In Poland, legal aid attorneys receive 120 Zloty—roughly this translates into $30 US for an entire case—at the first instance of a proceeding, which is at a district court. For representing claimants at the appeal court, they receive an additional 50 % of the lower court tariff. Consequently, lawyers often have to put a significant number of pro bono hours into involuntary-admission cases.

Moreover, attorneys frequently struggle to balance legal aid cases with the private practices from which they derive their living. Indeed, such cases imposed mandatorily on attorneys in Poland can constitute up to 20 % of an attorney's entire legal practice. Although some lawyers are able, willing, and have the resources to take seriously their legal aid responsibility in involuntary-admission cases, this in spite of the low remuneration and a significant commitment of time and energy; others perform only the bare minimum required by law—purporting only to *advocate* for their "clients."

A. Doll (✉)
University of Victoria, Victoria, BC, Canada
e-mail: amzajaczkowska2@gmail.com

© The Editor(s) (if applicable) and The Author(s) 2016
B. Burstow (ed.), *Psychiatry Interrogated*,
DOI 10.1007/978-3-319-41174-3_10

Further contributing to the conundrum is the fact that it is almost impossible to challenge any arguments put forward by psychiatric "experts." Moreover, many lawyers feel that judges dismiss the work they put into these cases, both in preparing and in delivering "sound" arguments. Advocacy for their clients' interests that involves new facts and evidence puts them in conflict with the court, which prioritizes quick adjudication of involuntary-admission cases. Correspondingly, departure from the judicially set role of a "figurant" carries adverse consequences.

All of which—even for those lawyers committed to their legal aid duties—only adds to the already burdensome nature of the work. The key issue here is that the involuntarily admitted—that is, *the very persons who need spirited lawyering*—may not receive appropriate advocacy. In this context, a right to representation, a key guarantee of "due process" under the inherently coercive procedure of involuntary admission, may be nothing more than a formalistic legal institution with no substantive meaning.

This story of lawyering for involuntarily confined people is told from the perspective of lawyers in order to shed light on the "experiences of clients and lawyers in concrete legal contexts" (Bellow and Minow 1996, p. 1) and to provide a firsthand account of the workings and limitations of the law and legal institutions. The objective of this chapter is not to defend lawyers or the quality of their work, especially as these can vary. Nor is it to address lawyers' attitudes toward their involuntarily committed "clients" and their often uncritical acceptance of the concept of "mental illness," which can also be troublesome. Rather, the objective here is to present a fuller picture of lawyering in cases deemed of lesser importance for attorneys and judges and to illustrate how this marginal position of involuntary-admission cases is operationalized by means of various "boss texts" organizing legal aid in Poland. Of particular significance are the Polish Mental Health Act of 1994 (MHA 1994) and the 2002 Ministry of Justice's Decree on Tariffs for Attorneys and Responsibility of the State Treasury for Unpaid Legal Aid Fees (Decree of Ministry of Justice, September 28, 2002).

This chapter shows how social relations embedded in legal and executive texts organize the everyday work of legal aid lawyers involved in involuntary-admission cases. Because these cases tend to be relegated to the margins of lawyers' work, it will be argued that these features of the legal aid system determine how much effort lawyers put into them. When explained in a systematic way, law stories provide not only "insights into how the legal workers and those affected by law make their choices, understand their actions, and experience the frustrations and satisfactions they entail" (Bellow and Minow 1996, p. 1) but also reveal institutional priorities that organize/restrain those choices and actions.

The basis for this discussion is an institutional ethnographic study conducted by the author over a period of 18 months (between August 2012 and February 2014) in Polish psychiatric hospitals and courts. The study included extensive observation at those sites, numerous interviews with legal and psychiatric professionals and staff, informal conversations, and extended analysis of laws and legal and administrative documents. Institutional ethnography (IE) was the main approach (Smith 2005, 2006) and was particularly suitable for this endeavor. Its focus is on people's engagement with institutional complexes and how this engagement shapes the experiences of individuals receiving and/ or providing services. IE takes professional concerns seriously, grounded in the practical experience of working in the healthcare and legal systems (or the not-for-profit sector), about what does not work for the people they serve.

While IE explores people's everyday experiences and the disjuncture between people's needs or intentions and what institutions offer (Smith 2005), and while other pieces in this particular anthology begin by looking at the disjuncture for "clients" and survivors, in IE, professional workers also can be approached as sites of disjuncture. Insofar as professional workers are the location of the disjuncture, investigations of this ilk link the "troubles" of professionals to the specific features of systems and their trans-local organization, showing how the working of the system constrains the ability of professionals to best support their "clients" or "patients" (Rankin and Campbell 2006). That is precisely the intent of this chapter's study.

I begin my discussion with an overview of the Polish Mental Health Act of 1994 concerning the regulation of involuntary admission and the procedural rights regime, with an emphasis on the right to representation.

POLAND'S INVOLUNTARY-ADMISSION PROCEDURE

In Poland, the Mental Health Act of 1994 (MHA 1994, Ch. 3) regulates involuntary admissions to psychiatric facilities. That MHA established substantive grounds for involuntary admission and a procedural framework for issuing and controlling the legality of involuntary-admission decisions. Involuntary admission is an inherently violent procedure, featuring, as it does, seriously uneven power relations between psychiatrists and admitted persons. In Poland and elsewhere, reformers involved in mental health reforms envisioned procedural rights as remedies, at least to some extent, to the power imbalance and saw them as contributing to the well-being of "patients" (Dabrowski and Kubicki 1994; Arben 1999). Reformers thought that "[s]ubstantive improvements in the lot of the mentally disordered would follow from a recognition of their rights" (Rose 1986, p. 177).

Equipped with procedural rights, "patients" of psychiatric institutions were seen to be in a position to "demand and obtain" their substantive rights accordingly (Rose 1986). For example, a "patient" could challenge the legality of an admission decision pertaining to the commitment. For substantive and procedural rights were precisely there to ensure that nobody is kept confined in psychiatric institutions "illegally." The Polish Mental Health Act of 1994 was enacted after more than 20 years of meticulous work drafting and legislating it. It introduced a system of legal control over admission decisions that is more extensive than that seen in other jurisdictions (Burstow 2015; Carver 2011).

First, the 1994 MHA introduced a strict time frame for psychiatrists to decide about involuntary admission and subsequently for the reviewing of those decisions by an "independent" judicial body. Within 72 hours of involuntary admission, the director of a psychiatric facility needs to notify a district court about it. Within the next 48 hours, a district court judge from the court's family division is obligated to come to the facility and meet with the admitted person. If the judge finds no grounds for recommending a discharge of the committed person from the facility (because of unmet substantive grounds for an involuntary admission), the case goes for a full review to a district court at a courthouse. The hearing needs to be held within two weeks of the judge's visitation.

Second, the Act ratified a comprehensive legal framework for controlling admission decisions. As Figure 10.1 shows, the admission decision is reviewed by at least one, potentially two, courts at least twice (by the lower court) and once (by the upper court) in addition to a review conducted by the supervisor of the psychiatric facility. The Act ratifies two types of review: (1) a system of mandatory review of all involuntary-admission decisions by a supervising authority of the facility, by a district court judge, and by a district court in the

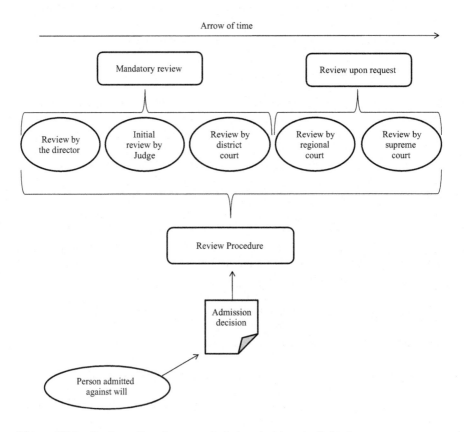

Figure 10.1   Review of involuntary-admission decisions in Poland

jurisdiction of the hospital; (2) a system of review by an upper court that is undertaken upon the "patient's" motion. Finally, the appeal decision can be reviewed in the form of a *cassation* document submitted to the Supreme Court of Poland.

Third, the MHA 1994 and provisions of Polish civil procedure ratified that a "patient", is a party to this controlling procedure and thus is guaranteed all the rights accorded to such a party. Specifically, the person has rights such as: to participate in case hearings, to make claims, to submit new evidence, to respond to evidence provided by the opposing party, and to appeal the lower court decision. A person can undertake all of these activities personally or through an appointed representative. Thus, a right to representation (i.e., an extension of a person's privilege to exercise his or her legal rights) emerges as a significant aspect of "due process" in Poland, a breach of which can invalidate the entire legal proceeding in a case.

In the next section, I will show that in their realization of these procedural rights, persons who are involuntarily committed to psychiatric facilities in Poland heavily rely on legal assistance provided by legal aid attorneys. This is due to the particular circumstances in which they find themselves.

Access to Legal Representation in Involuntary-Admission Cases

Involuntary psychiatric admission is an emergency event that may catch people by surprise. People are thus often financially unprepared and are frequently entirely unaware of their need for a lawyer. Hiring a lawyer requires resources, which the admitted person may not have at her disposal or may not have with her in the ward. Yet, retaining a lawyer in Poland typically necessitates upfront payment for legal service.[2]

Even when the admitted person has the financial resources necessary, there are several barriers to accessing them when one is locked in a closed ward. Confinement in such a place significantly curtails a person's contact with the outside world, including access to banks and ATMs. For instance, in the psychiatric facility where I conducted my research, a bank and an ATM machine are located in hospital lounges or outside of the building, inaccessible to psychiatric patients. Moreover, the confined person would need permission to leave the ward; however, such permission is not given to anyone viewed as aggressive or deemed an escape risk, which is a common assumption about those admitted involuntarily.

For other medically related instances, family may facilitate access to financial resources if needed; however, in the context of involuntary admission, family members tend to be less helpful because they have often initiated the involuntary hospitalization in question. According to my research, the only case in which a lawyer of choice was willing to step in without advanced payment was when the admitted person had an ongoing relationship with that lawyer, or that lawyer had represented her in other cases.

In Poland, any person who cannot afford to hire a lawyer can ask for legal aid representation.[3] Still, the person must demonstrate that he does not have the financial resources to hire a lawyer. This is not true, though, for proceedings that fall under the scope of the MHA of 1994. These are "cost-exempted," meaning that neither is a filing fee charged for starting a legal action (e.g., submitting an appeal) nor is legal aid conditional on the financial needs of the requesting person.

This, along with less formal requirements for document submission, is supposed to facilitate access to justice for civilly committed persons given the precarious context in which they find themselves. Nonetheless, lawyers' participation in civil commitment procedures is minimal. I encountered only rare instances where committed persons appointed the lawyer of their choice, or requested a legal aid lawyer, regardless of their financial means. One significant factor related to the low frequency of attorney appointments became clear during my research: Involuntarily admitted persons are often confused about the nature of their admission, its duration, and its possible consequences. Instead of seeing court involvement as a practice that is to "guarantee" their rights, a judge's visit to the hospital for the initial assessment tends only to further confuse the admitted persons.

What I noticed, additionally, is that even when the committed person requests a lawyer, this information does not necessarily reach the decision-making authority responsible for such an appointment. For example, a field note stated:

[A] young woman was admitted without consent to a psychiatric facility. Since the very beginning, she was vocal that she disagreed with the admission and that she was going to challenge it by legal means. She was aware of both of the grounds, which need to be met for an involuntary admission, and of her procedural rights. She informed her leading doctor that she would like to consult a lawyer and asked for one. Yet, the doctor never passed this request to the court that makes the decision in that matter. Nor did the judge who came to meet her note her request in her patient files. The woman was not appointed a lawyer until she once again requested one, this time in writing, directly submitted to the court. In the meantime, however, the hearing proceeded and the lower court adjudicated the case. She was granted the lawyer only after she submitted an appeal, and after she had been discharged from the hospital by a medical authority.

Although this finding cannot be generalized, persons who tend to request legal aid lawyers are those familiar with the legal system. Through their education, work, or previous admissions, they have knowledge of their rights regardless of whether a judge informs them. They may, however, still struggle to access legal aid.

In general, I have not witnessed a single judge providing meaningful information to "patients" about the nature of the legal procedure, not to mention the total lack of information provided to involuntarily admitted persons about their right to professional representation. Indeed, the admitted persons may not even be aware that a lawyer's help and assistance is available to them.

Nonetheless, one of the key guarantees of a patient's right to representation stems from the MHA of 1994, Art. 48:

The Court can appoint a legal aid lawyer, for a person whom the procedure concerns, even if the person does not request it, but due to her mental health the person is not capable of submitting such a request, yet the court conceives lawyer's participation as necessary.

Thus, a judge is obligated to appoint a lawyer for a civilly committed person who is unable to undertake his or her own representation. Yet, district judges tend to apply this article narrowly limiting such an appointment to two kinds of situations, when:

(a) According to a psychiatric assessment the person is "incapable" to consent to an admission and thus participate in the procedure consciously; or
(b) The admitted person is less than 16 years old.

In these two instances, the MHA of 1994 requires a "supported" decision-making procedure for which the presence of a lawyer is mandatory. Otherwise, the judge risks the decision being overturned on appeal on the grounds of invalidity of the proceeding—specifically that the admitted person was deprived of the privilege to defend her rights. In the preceding instances, an admitted person needs to have a legal representative acting on her behalf to ensure validity of control of the involuntary admission decision. Indeed, those appointments are the most common when it comes to legal aid representation in the context of an involuntary admission procedure.

A judge also can appoint a lawyer in any involuntary-admission case when she or he recognizes that *participation of a legal professional in the case is necessary*. Yet, here the matter of priorities becomes clearly visible, as well as the gap between the practice as it happens at actual local sites and the Polish Supreme Court's recommendation for such a practice. The disparity between the right to legal aid representation for persons who cannot participate and what actually happens in practice will become clearer as the chapter proceeds. For the time being, suffice it to say that district court judges predominantly appoint legal aid lawyers in situations where they are required by law to do so. This is in spite of the Supreme Court's recommendation for treating legal representation as a mandatory element of a "due" review procedure of an involuntary admission decision (Supreme Court... in II CZ 2/12, 2012).

Although recent decisions of the Supreme Court are problematic in some aspects because the Court represents a formalist take on the issue of legal representation, ignoring its reality and promoting representation over patient's participation—their significance lies in the recognition that patients face multiple barriers in realizing their procedural rights. Existence of these barriers renders legal assistance necessary. In actuality, legal aid lawyers are commonly not appointed until the case reaches the appeal stage.

The next two sections discuss two features of legal aid services in Poland that significantly determine how much time and energy lawyers can and are willing to put into involuntary-admission cases.

LEGAL AID IN POLAND

Although marginal in number, legal aid representation still predominates in involuntary-admission cases. Yet, attorneys perceive legal aid cases as distinct from other legal work because of their mandatory character, the urgency of the action required of a lawyer, the potential mismatch between the scope of the case and attorneys' specializations, and the low remuneration. It is important to understand how this legal representation is organized as being distinct from other types of lawyers' work to reveal implications of this organization. What follows, accordingly, is a discussion of: (1) the mandatory and urgent character of these legal aid appointments as well as their inconsideration of lawyers' specialization and (2) the internal hierarchy of legal aid cases that affects lawyer's remuneration for legal aid work.

"Forced" Cause Lawyering

In Poland, legal aid service is mandatory and as such, contributes to lawyers' experiences of seeing it as burdensome—an unwelcome duty. Every practicing attorney and in-house council is obligated to take legal aid cases in addition to his or her private practice (Bar Law 1982). Attorneys are duty-bound to provide quality representation, for which they are professionally and financially responsible. This leaves no room for professional choice and voluntarism based on a personal and/or moral commitment to a case or its cause. An attorney generally cannot refuse a legal aid case because of insufficient time or a scheduling conflict with other hearings. The only justifiable grounds on which an attorney can refuse a legal aid appointment is in cases of a conflict of interest—for instance, where the lawyer has represented or advised or is representing the opposing party.

Once the lawyer is appointed, he or she is immediately duty-bound and the appointment continues for the duration of the case, including any appeal. Civil commitment cases, more often than other types of legal aid cases, may require a lawyer to take action immediately. Interviewed attorneys reported facing certain difficulties in providing quality lawyering in such cases while maintaining the regular workload integral to their private practices.

To accommodate this mandatory duty, appointed attorneys often need to make significant adjustments to their regular workload; this is possible when lawyers do not carry extensive private practices, or in those instances where they do but have help from articled students. Still, the work attorneys face in negotiating mandatory lawyering in legal aid cases, and specifically in civil commitment cases, requires a significant amount of time and attention, which presents them with an equally significant challenge in trying to make a living out of lawyering.

Moreover, legal aid appointments, at least at the level of a district court, have an urgent quality. Because civil commitment cases are structured around tight deadlines, the appointed lawyer generally begins work immediately. Right away, she is faced with tight time frames that require psychiatric and legal work within the first week of a person's admission to ensure that nobody is kept confined unnecessarily or illegally. Most commonly, judges appoint lawyers after the initial hospital visit, or when the "patient" submits an appeal that reaches the appeal court. This appointment procedure, however, requires coordination and interaction between a court and a local bar because the bar council holds the power to assign an individual lawyer to a case. Given that, the time between the court's appointment decision and the hearing date may be less than two weeks. If this is added to the time needed for the appointment procedure at the bar council and for notification, the appointed lawyer may have as little as two days to prepare for a hearing.

Given the considerable urgency of civil commitment cases, the appointed lawyer may not be able to participate in the hearing because of a scheduling conflict. Some lawyers report having as many as six legal aid cases scheduled for the same day and approximate time. In this situation, the appointed lawyer needs to find a substitute lawyer who can appear in her stead. This usually requires several phone calls, delivering of case files to the substitute, and often providing remuneration out of her own pocket. Along with tariffs accepted in a community, in fact a one-time substitution at a hearing may cost more than what the appointed lawyer will receive from the government for providing representation in the entire involuntary-admission case.

The suddenness of appointments is not the only problem for lawyers faced with trying to merge them with their regular workloads. Another issue is the utter lack of attention paid to a lawyer's specialization. Because appointments in civil commitment cases are assigned randomly from a list, a lawyer's field of specialization becomes irrelevant to the procedure.[4] Adding to the problem is the fact that, in Poland, attorneys are not typically trained in mental health law, nor are there many who specialize in this field.

This means that appointees require additional time to prepare for cases that they may encounter only on very rare occasions. For instance, the lawyers I interviewed had been involved in as few as one, or at most several involuntary-committed cases in their professional careers. This, in combination with tight deadlines and the marginal position of these cases in attorneys' overall practices, contributes to the mistaken perception that civil commitment cases are unproblematic and straightforward. One consequence is that, while lawyers were ostensibly representing the interests of their clients, they were in fact— perhaps unintentionally—utterly silencing their clients' voices. To understand more fully how this happens, these challenges need to be placed in the broader context of recent neoliberal changes to the organization of lawyers' work.

The economic relations in which a lawyer's work is embedded and to which it responds, contribute to the relegation of civil commitment cases to the margins of lawyers' work (within which private cases occupy the principal position). Since the mid-2000s, legal professionals in Poland, specifically attorneys and in-house councils, have undergone a significant professional shift because of the opening of their profession to a greater number of law graduates. Because of these changes, between 2004 and 2013 the number of attorneys in Poland increased from about 6000 to almost 13,000 practicing attorneys.[5] With that increase, the general pauperization of Polish society, and broader access to online legal services and legal information, many lawyers find themselves struggling, in the face of financial difficulties, to uphold their private practices. Given these changes, fierce competition for clients becomes an everyday reality for lawyers, who are often forced to decrease fees to make themselves more competitive and to seek more cases to meet their financial needs.[6] Thus, to ensure financial stability, or even sometimes to simply maintain their practices, many lawyers prioritize cases that are financially profitable and allocate their time and energy accordingly.

Working for "Free" or Money for "Nothing"?

While attorneys treat state-appointed lawyering as a fulfillment of their public service obligation, Bar Law 1982, some cases are less welcome than others. Whether an attorney feels his work is adequately remunerated and his arguments are adequately heard plays an important role in how the attorney experiences legal aid cases and, more broadly, the amount of work he does as a lawyer. Involuntary-admission cases are located at the far end of this spectrum as they involve a significant time commitment.

Remuneration for attorneys' work in Poland is regulated by the Ministry of Justice's Decree on Tariffs for Attorneys and Responsibility of the State Treasury for Unpaid Legal Aid Fees (Ministry of Justice, 28 September 2002). Once the 1964 "Code of Civil Procedure" determined how to distribute the costs of proceedings between parties, the 2002 Decree on attorney's fees set up how much a winning party would be reimbursed for legal representation, for example. For cases in which a legal aid lawyer was appointed to represent a party, the 2002 Decree regulates how much the attorney will be paid for the work. Because determination of costs is an integral part of any legal decision in Poland, judges refer to the 2002 Decree on attorneys' tariffs on a daily basis.

Although on the surface the 2002 Decree appears to be a technical act ratifying tariffs, it does far more than that. It performs an important piece of ideological work that organizes how judges practice law, how much attention they pay to specific cases, and how lawyers' work in those cases is valued and accordingly reimbursed. The point here is, the 2002 Decree on attorneys' fees constructs involuntary-admission cases as less important and the attorney's work put into those cases of no value unless it aligns with priorities held by judges.

Next I will show how this 2002 Decree established a hierarchy of cases, of work, and of knowledge—and consequently contributes to the marginalization of involuntary-admission cases in lawyers' practices. Specifically, the Decree's paragraphs 4.1 and 4.2, as well as paragraph 19, are essential in organizing legal aid lawyering in involuntary-admission cases as marginal. They are discussed in the following section.

Hierarchy of Cases

Paragraph 4.1 of the 2002 Decree directly sets the framework for the practice for delineation of cases and placing them in a hierarchical order by differentiating attorneys' tariffs according to types of cases. It reads:

Cases are remunerated according to the value of an object or a service under litigation, or a type of case, or value of claim in court execution proceedings.

Thus, there are two groupings of cases for the purpose of remuneration. In cases, such as torts, contract-related claims, and court execution proceedings, the remuneration that lawyers will receive is decided based on the value of object/service criteria. In all other cases the remuneration is based on the case type (e.g., whether it is a custody case, an incapacitation case, etc.).

There are significant disparities in remuneration for the two distinct groupings of cases. Cases related to the protection of goods and rights related to market economy are at the top of the case hierarchy and, accordingly, lawyer's tariffs are the highest in those cases. Correspondingly, cases related to patents or other types of intellectual property, which are important to a competitive liberal market—although placed in the second grouping of cases—are still assigned higher tariffs than, for example, family law cases in the same groupings.

Now, for attorney services in cases where the value of the exchange object exceeds Zl 200,000 (around $70,000 US), an attorney would receive remuneration that is as much as *60 times* higher than what she would receive for services in a civil commitment case. Because the 2002 Decree does not ratify fees, mental health law cases *are not directly specified in the act* (par. 5). Thus, by convention, courts in this situation apply the fee assigned for the most similar case. Commonly, judges apply a fee for *other undefined cases*, and this fee is Zl 120 —around $40 US. Lower fees are typically applied to civil commitment cases, and more generally to cases that deal with personal liberties (e.g., incapacitation).

This hierarchy of tariffs creates a hierarchy of importance. The cases for which remuneration is higher are constructed in this text as more important and more complicated. Not surprisingly, those cases ranked toward the top of the tariff hierarchy tend to be more welcomed by legal aid lawyers as they are better remunerated than those cases lower on the scale (e.g., involuntary-admission cases). The internal hierarchy of cases established by the Decree places involuntary-admission cases—the very ones that need spirited lawyering—at the bottom of the hierarchy, which directly influences how much lawyers receive for their services.

HIERARCHY OF WORK

Paragraph 2.1 of the 2002 Decree further shapes the ideological foundation of the text by setting a causal link between the hierarchy of cases and the work needed to protect certain goods/rights. This section is located at the beginning of the Decree, before specific fees are even listed. It provides a discursive frame for reading the following articles of the Decree, including articles specifying legal tariffs. Paragraph 2.1 reads:

> *Deciding upon the remuneration for a lawyer for the representation, court takes into consideration necessary labor input of the attorney, nature of the case, and attorneys' input in the resolution of the case.*

This paragraph fosters an assumption that tariffs assigned for specific cases that are listed in Chapters 3–5 of the Decree are an adequate remuneration for the activities involved in lawyering in those cases as they take into account complexity and the "nature" of them. Subsequently, the necessary labor input in lawyering in a case is constructed accordingly.

The 2002 Decree on attorney's tariffs established a presumption that the complexity of cases is related to the value of the subject matter. Yet, the implications of this presumption are enormous for lawyers and their "clients." By setting the frame as they do for the necessary amount of work involved in cases, all other work activities undertaken are rendered invisible and subsequently disregarded. As a result, all those activities that are not seen by a judge as a necessary labor input remain unpaid. The point here is that provisions in the Decree guide judges in determining what is considered necessary labor input, while overlooking the actual amount of work needed for quality of service. As such, the Decree provides a direct link between the fees and the complexity ("the nature") of the case in a way that structures involuntary-admission cases as less important and not involving a significant amount of work because the tariff applied as adequate to these cases is around $30 US. To understand the extent of the disparity, it is important to take into account the actual activities needed to provide proper legal representation in such cases.

Although the amount of work involved in the representation can vary depending on the precise timing of an appointment, it includes many interconnected activities. The result is that the actual amount of work legal aid lawyers put toward good lawyering stands in stark contrast with the 2002 Decree's scheme of remuneration. For a lawyer appointed at the district court stage, work may involve participation in a number of hearings, meeting with a "client," collecting case documents, writing an appeal, participating in appeal hearing(s), waiting for those hearings, and so forth. The amount of work in cases for which an attorney would receive $30 US may not differ, sometimes may even exceed the amount of work necessary for lawyering in cases remunerated at 60 times more.

Nevertheless, activities that are not undertaken in front of the court, but are integral to lawyering (e.g., reading court files), are invisible to the judges who handle lawyers' remuneration. They are invisible because the institutional discourse embedded in the 2002 Decree constructs a judge's consciousness in such a way as to reflect the priority of Poland's legal system. It sets specific tenets of remuneration and guides the attention of judges to interpret lawyers' legal aid representation work not only very narrowly but also according to economic and formalistic priorities, oriented toward the functioning of the juridical system in Poland.

HIERARCHY OF INPUT

The 2002 Decree on attorneys' tariffs further opens space for regulating attorneys' legal work, along with the state's financial and ideological interests, through equipping judges with the discretionary power to determine whether a lawyer contributed to the resolution of the case, and which kind of input justifies an increase in remuneration for her. Based on this determination, a judge can increase the minimal fee set for a case if the judge decides that the fee is not adequate to *the labor input of an attorney, the nature of the case, and attorney's input in the resolution of the case.* Paragraph 2.2 reads:

> *The basis for remuneration for attorneys' service [...] is the minimal tariff listed in [the Decree's] Chapters 3–5. This remuneration cannot be higher than six fold of the minimal tariff nor it can exceed the value of the case.*

Additionally, Paragraph 19 specifies the increase of the minimal tariffs in regards to legal aid representation. It reads:

> *Unpaid expenditure for a legal aid service is covered by the State Treasure and this expenditure includes:*

> *(1) Remuneration in the amount up to 150 % of the minimal tariff listed in [the Decree's] Chapters 3–5.*
> *(2) Necessary and documented expenses of an attorney.*

The preceding listed provisions related to the potential increase in an attorney's fee are troublesome for at least three reasons.

First, by setting up this strict limit to which tariffs can be increased, the Decree still allows very low remuneration in cases that are located at the bottom of the hierarchy of importance. Second, it directly devalues the work even more when the work is pursued as legal aid work. Third, the Decree legitimizes the judge's decision as to what kind of contribution, and further, knowledge is valuable in the context of legal proceeding. Accordingly, this creates a significant barrier for lawyers engaged in meaningful lawyering that aligns with their "clients'" interests.

The term "contribution to the resolution of the case," which guides a judge's assessment of the value of a lawyer's work, allows institutional priorities (e.g., procedural economy) to enter judicial practice and structure what is considered valuable input into the case and, more generally, what knowledge input is valued. Consequently, the lawyers that I interviewed reported that judges consistently dismiss well-grounded legal arguments when those arguments contest the legality of involuntary admission, specifically, and the psychiatric opinion that speaks to its legality. Indeed, judges tend to dismiss arguments advanced by lawyers, except in those cases when they point to formal problems already noted by judges. So for lawyers, it is challenging to engage in a meaningful representation of an involuntarily admitted person not only because of the courts' often uncritical reliance on psychiatric expert opinions but also because their attempts to engage are interpreted by judges as mere delaying tactics.

My data suggest that the practice of increasing lawyer's fees for work in involuntary-admission cases is nonexistent. On the contrary, judges believe that even this $30 US is more than what lawyers deserve for their work. They see lawyer's work as participation in a "5-minute" court hearing (*sic!*). This speaks to the mistaken perception, shared among judges, that attorneys get "money for nothing." What goes along with this, because commitment cases are structured in such a way as to be of lesser importance in the hierarchy of legal protection, and assumed uncomplicated, any attempt of a lawyer to contest some of the "scientific" "facts" is treated by judges as "unnecessary prolongation of a case" that rather should be punished not remunerated (Figure 10.2).

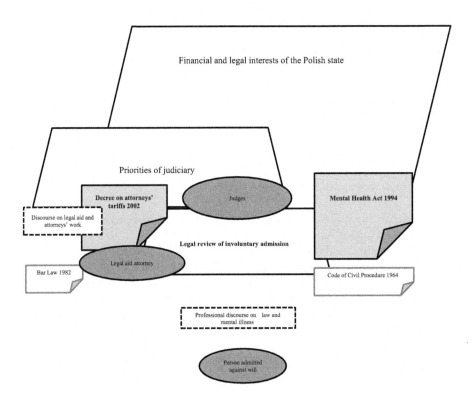

Figure 10.2 Organization of legal aid lawyering in involuntary-admission cases in Poland

LAWYERING FOR THE "MAD"

This section follows an actual legal aid case to see what legal aid representation *really* involves. It will become clearly visible how the textually mediated practices of judges and the organization of the legal aid system in Poland, instead of fostering the quality of lawyering received by involuntarily admitted persons, in fact impedes it. The case also illustrates how inadequate the Polish system of legal aid is in encouraging lawyers to undertake and pursue quality work. It also shows how lawyers and their clients' interests are subsumed under the interests and priorities of the judiciary and that of the state.

A young attorney was appointed as a legal aid lawyer for an involuntarily admitted person. The person had been assessed as "suffering from a mental illness" and as posing a "danger to others," specifically to his family. The lawyer was appointed only after the committed person had submitted an appeal. Thus, the lawyer's representation involved preparation before and participation at the appeal hearing. This appeal submitted by the "client" had formal deficiencies and so the lawyer was obligated to fix them. The appeal was not professionally written. The lawyer's task was to correct the defects and to prove all facts supporting the client's stance. Along with the civil procedure, the attorney was given seven days to correct the formal defects. The case required urgent intervention.

First, the attorney went to the court to read case files. He became familiar with the case. Then he drove to the hospital to meet with his client, whereupon he learned that the "client" did not want to be in the hospital. The client also provided him with new information that contextualized the moment and events that led to the admission. On the basis of the information so gleaned, the attorney prepared a draft of a motion with new facts and evidence. Then he went back to the client to consult about the accuracy of this draft. After gaining his client's approval, the attorney submitted the document to the court. This all consumed a lot of time. On the hearing date, he participated in the hearing in the absence of his client for the person had not been transported to the courthouse. He was thus the only one there to defend his client's interest and represent his stance. The judge went on to dismiss the appeal. For all the work that he did for the case, the attorney received $30 US.

This case clearly speaks to the amount of work needed to do meaningful and engaged lawyering and to the inadequacy of the remuneration, and it highlights the inherent contradiction—that judges see only those activities they personally can observe; namely, presence at the hearing and submission of a document. The point here is, often lawyers' work is only understood in terms of how many hearings they participate in or how many documents they submit. Yet, as this case makes clear, there is a huge spectrum of activities that are integral to lawyering that are rendered invisible to judges. In this case, these activities included, for example: "reading case files," "meeting with the client," "preparing documents for court submission," and so forth. Moreover, what is crucial to understand here, general terms (e.g., "reading files") consist of a broad spectrum of other activities that are subsumed under those terms, all these made and constructed as "nonexistent."

Take as an example the activity of "reading files." This term, in lawyers' parlance, covers all of the intermediate steps necessary just to get to the point of actually reading files. First, one needs to arrange with court staff a time and date for obtaining files. This requires making a phone call to determine whether the files are in the courthouse, and then scheduling a time with the courthouse's reading room. Sometimes attorneys need to call several times to schedule this reading because the files may be circulating between court staff and judges. Making notes on case files or making photocopies requires additional time. Even though a number of attorneys currently use their own digital cameras to photocopy file documents, some still rely on the court to copy documents for them. In the latter instance, they need to schedule a pick-up time for those photocopies and then physically retrieve them.

On top of all that, there is the actual reading of the text files; extracting evidence and facts; making strategic decisions about the case; and deciding what needs to be elaborated on, which challenges to bring, and what new evidence to present to the judge. These activities comprise, and are enmeshed in, the process of "reading files." Thus, there is a significant discrepancy between what is viewed as indispensable work involved in lawyering in civil commitment cases and what happens in real life, or how much lawyers need to do for the cases.

In addition to activities related to the preparation of legal documents, legal aid attorneys need to participate in court hearings. In criminal cases, they are paid for attending each hearing, *over and above their base case fee*; however, in civil commitment cases lawyers are paid *only the base fee* regardless of how many mandatory hearings may occur. A lawyer's participation in hearings additionally involves other time-consuming activities. Polish courts are notoriously in a constant state of delay. According to a report prepared in 2014 by the non-profit Court Watch Poland Foundation, such delays usually range between 30 minutes and three hours (Pilitowski and Burdziej 2013/2014). This time is usually spent, or rather wasted, in a hallway in front of the courtroom. Time spent waiting for the hearing counts as part of the lawyer's work on that specific case, as he or she obviously cannot engage in work on any other. Thus, the term "participation in a hearing" renders invisible all activities that require time and effort (e.g., waiting). When we take into account all those activities involved in actual lawyering, we see quite a different picture of a lawyer's work than what is constructed by judges practicing using the 2002 Decree.

What further complicates the picture, the amount of time and energy lawyers can and are willing to give to these cases, depends on the workload they face in their regular practices. Note, in this regard, the following interchange that I had with an attorney during an interview on February 10, 2013:

> *Agnieszka:* Given what you told me at this interview, that that legal aid case was at the beginning of your legal career, as a more seasoned attorney with more clients, would you be able to engage to that same extent if you got this case now?

> *Attorney:* I think that now I would limit myself to only one visit. This is because those cases require a lot of time. Yet, everything depends on the stage of the legal procedure to which I would be appointed.

Although in the case just presented, the attorney performed a significant amount of work and made an effort to meet with his "client," many attorneys predominately rely on case documents while pursuing representation of their legal aid clients. This carries an inherent danger of marginalizing the voices of those they are supposed to represent. For example, one attorney interviewee, whose engagement in the case could not be questioned because he devoted significant time and effort to his lawyering, stated:

> I did not need [to see] the client to defend his rights. I think that arguments that I formulated [based on case files] were sufficient (January 22, 2013).

Despite the fact that lawyers with sufficient time may visit the patient in the hospital, those who do not, or cannot incorporate such a visit into their regular workload, rely on their clients' textual representations put together in case documents. This, of course, has a direct and negative impact on the person being represented, particularly as it affects what can be known about her. It is important to point out here that, in general, hearings are held in a courthouse in the absence of the committed person. Thus, attorneys' detailed knowledge of their clients and the circumstances of admission are crucial—something seriously compromised if such visits never take place. I would add too that the above-mentioned lawyer was not even aware that his client's rights were violated in another way—that is, all the correspondence was sent to an incorrect address, preventing him from participating in the hearing concerning his client on a personal level.

This case also makes visible the disparity of assessing lawyers' work through the judicially informed notion of the "contribution to the resolution of the case." The young lawyer clearly provided essential facts and evidence that should have been considered as an important contribution to the resolution of the case as he contextualized the facts of his "client's" admission. For example, he provided information regarding the context and the nature of so deemed "aggressive" and "dangerous" behavior of his client, which happened in the context of a family dispute. Correspondingly, in an effort to prove the facts of his case, the lawyer issued a request to call witnesses present at the incident. Yet a court, without an explanation of the decision's rationale, rejected his motion. Besides the unfavorable consequences and what this shows about the short shrift given the rights of involuntarily committed persons, this example speaks to the low status, which is intimately connected with low remuneration and lack of recognition of work, afforded lawyers in such cases.

By contrast, the value of the contribution of "experts" is clearly demonstrated through the system of remuneration for their opinions. Contrary to the way lawyers are treated, experts appointed by courts are paid by the number of hours of work spent on the production of their opinions, and those hours may include all the necessary activities that precede them (Grabowska et al. 2014). Moreover, the amount claimed by experts is taken for granted by judges (even when their remuneration is very high) and hardly ever reassessed, which makes it very difficult for that expenditure to be contested by parties to the case.

These are a few of the barriers that constrain meaningful engagement of a legal aid lawyer in lawyering for civilly committed people in Poland.

Concluding Remarks

As can now be clearly seen, the procedures surrounding a legal aid appointment and remuneration for legal aid lawyers' work relocates legal aid civil commitment cases to the margins of attorneys' work. To ensure that the right to legal representation has meaning and is not a mere formality, conditions of work involved in legal aid in Poland need to change. First, the system of appointment and remuneration needs to be altered. Lawyers also need more time to critically engage in those cases that are not prioritized by the Polish state. Specifically, in those cases regarding personal liberty and bodily integrity, such as involuntary-admission cases, people need spirited lawyering. Those cases are much more complex than even lawyers initially tend to perceive them and how judges treat them.

What goes along with this, to allow lawyers to deliver quality service, which is a key element of substantive justice, the state cannot shift the costs of legal aid onto the shoulders of attorneys and take advantage of their provision of an obligatory public service. Too often in public discourse, attorneys' work is construed as a public service they are compelled to undertake despite low remuneration. Contrary to what the Polish Constitutional Tribunal (Constitutional Tribunal in Ts 263/13, 2013) has insinuated, attorneys are not "missionaries," and their "cause" lawyering is a work that deserves adequate remuneration.

Moreover, as with other experts, lawyers appointed by state authority to undertake certain tasks should be remunerated for *all the activities* this job involves. Instead of assuming that cases (e.g., an involuntary-commitment case) require less work, lawyers should be given an opportunity to bill for the time actually spent on these cases. This is accepted legal practice for any other experts. Thus, remuneration should be altered to make it hour-based, not case-based.

Finally, the system of mandatory work is an oppressive one and does not ensure quality legal service. It undermines lawyers' choice to engage in legal aid work willingly and for the cause in which they believe. Furthermore, as an imposed obligation that stands in conflict with lawyers' legal practices, legal aid cases, specifically those located toward the bottom of the hierarchy, tend to be marginalized and usually do not receive the attention they need. Although it is beyond the scope of this chapter to provide an exact solution, clearly a change that allows for choice is necessary.

In the absence of such changes, the lawyer suffers. And what goes along with this, in the absence of such changes, despite the discourse of rights, the involuntarily committed person will continue to have compromised representation. Hopefully, more IE work will be done in this area. All being well, the study that figures in this chapter, the chapter itself, and future work of this ilk will set the stage for a sorely needed reevaluation.[7]

NOTES

1. Although legal aid service attorneys and in-house council are equally obligated as professional groups, I focus here (as I did in my research) on attorneys and their legal aid service because they are proximately appointed to deliver legal aid service, at least in civil commitment cases. On the Adwokatura Polska Blog (see http://www.adwokatura.pl/), it has been reported that the ratio of obligatory annual legal aid lawyers' cases to the number of cases taken on by in-house council is around 20:1. Moreover, the specificity of the work of attorneys and in-house council differs. For example, an in-house council may work on a regular employment contract while an attorney in Poland cannot.

2. Legal fees are usually significantly higher than tariffs for professional representation of choice, suggested in the 2002 Decree on attorneys' tariffs. Therefore, depending on the complexity of the case and on the amount of work required, an attorney of choice tends to charge up to several times more than what is defined in the Decree for the type of case.

3. There is an ongoing discussion about whether the courts are the right system in which decisions about granting a claimant legal aid should be made. This is an important concern because certain political priorities (e.g., the focus on expedited case processing and budgetary restrains of courts) do influence whether a client or potential client receives, or is even informed about, his or her rights to legal aid representation. See http://www.adwokat-mierzejewska. pl/doc/Pomoc_prawna_z_urzedu.pdf (Anonymous n.d.).

4. In this way, an appointment in a civil or administrative case also diverges from one in a criminal case. It is more likely that a lawyer with a specialization in criminal law would be appointed to the case by the court because a different system of legal appointments exists for legal aid criminal cases. The main difference has to do with *which legal authority*, either a court or a local bar council, has the power to appoint an individual attorney. While in criminal cases, legal aid lawyers are retained by the criminal court, in the other types of cases the local bar council retains this power. Now, in criminal cases judges tend to appoint lawyers whom they know, and who have experience representing people in criminal cases. By contrast, in civil commitment cases (as well as in other noncriminal cases), the names of attorneys are drawn from a list.

5. See http://blog.naveo.pl/2014/07/11/prognozy-rynku-uslug-prawniczych/ (Sowinski and Sek 2014).

6. Antkowiak (2010) points out that legal services in Poland are provided not only by attorneys and in-house lawyers but also by financial advisers, executors, notaries, and patent experts. In 2010, this added about 25 % to the total number of legal professionals (the total number of attorneys and in-house lawyers). Yet, the duty of legal aid service is imposed on attorneys and in-house councils only.

7. *Note:* The author would like to point out that subsequent to the submission of this chapter, the 2002 Decree was substituted by a new decree that is to take effect in 2016 (Decree of the Ministry of Justice, 22 October 2015). The new Decree, alas, changes nothing with respect to remuneration for mental health cases.

References

Anonymous. (n.a). *Pomoc prawna z urzedu a prawo do sadu.* Retrieved on August 11, 2015, from http://www.adwokat-mierzejewska.pl/doc/Pomoc_prawna_z_urzedu.pdf

Antkowiak, P. (2010). *The end of legal professions in Europe—The case of Poland.* Retrieved August 11, 2015, from https://www.academia.edu/3357140/

Arben, P. (1999). A commentary: Why civil commitment laws don't work the way they're supposed to. *Journal of Sociology and Social Welfare, 26,* 61–70.

Bar Act. (1982). *The law on the advocates' profession.* Retrieved on December 7, 2105, from http://www.ccbe.eu/fileadmin/user_upload/NTCdocument/en_poland_law_on_adv1_1188889310.pdf

Bellow, G., & Minow, M. (Eds.) (1996). *Law stories.* Ann Arbor: University of Michigan Press.

Burstow, B. (2015). *Psychiatry and the business of madness: An ethical and epistemological accounting.* New York: Palgrave Macmillan.

Carver, P. (2011). Mental health law in Canada. In J. Downie, T. Caulfield, & C. Flood (Eds.), *Canadian health law and policy.* Markham: LexisNexis.

Code of Civil Procedure. (1964). *Act of 17 November 1964.* Retrieved December 6, 2015, from ww.uaipit.com/files/documentos/0000004939_Polonia_Ley_Arbitraje_Codigo_Proc_Civil.pdf

Constitutional Tribunal. (2013). Decision Ts 263/13.

Dabrowski, S., & Kubicki, L. (1994). *Ustawa o ochronie zdrowia psychicznego: Przeglad wazniejszych orzeczen.* Warszawa: Instytut Psychiatrii i Neurologii.

Decree of Ministry of Justice. (2002, 28 September). Decree concerning legal fees for attorneys and responsibility of State Treasury for the cost of state funded legal aid. *Journal of Laws.* Position 163, Item 1348. Retrieved in Polish from http://isap.sejm.gov.pl/DetailsServlet?id=WDU20021631348

Decree of the Ministry of Justice. (2015, 22 October). Decree concerning covering by State Treasury the cost of state funded legal aid delivered by attorney. *Journal of Laws.* Item 189. Retrieved in Polish from http://isap.sejm.gov.pl/DetailsServlet?id=WDU20150001801

Grabowska, B., Pietryka, A., & Wolny, M. (2014). *Biegli sadowi w Polsce.* Warszawa: Helsinska Fundacja Praw Czlowieka.

Mental Health Act (MHA). (1994). Ch. 3.

Pilitowski, B., & Burdziej, S. (2013/2014). *Raport: Obywatelski monitoring sadow.* Torun: Fundacja Court Watch Polska.

Rankin, J., & Campbell, M. (2006). *Managing to nurse: Inside Canada's health care reform.* Toronto: University of Toronto Press.

Rose, N. (1986). Law, rights, and psychiatry. In P. Miller & N. Rose (Eds.), *The power of psychiatry* (pp. 177–213). Cambridge: Polity Press.

Smith, D. (2005). *Institutional ethnography: A sociology for people.* Landham: Altamira Press.

Smith, D. (2006). *Institutional ethnography as practice.* Landham: Rowman and Littlefield.

Sowinski, R., & Sek, T. (2014). *Prognoza rynku uslug prawniczych.* Retrieved in Polish August 11, 2015, from http://blog.naveo.pl/2014/07/11/prognozy-rynku-uslug-prawniczych/

Supreme Court of Poland. (2012). *Decision II CZ 2/12.*

CHAPTER 11

By Any Other Name: An Exploration of the Academic Development of Torture and Its Links to the Military and Psychiatry

Efrat Gold

I began my postsecondary education as an idealistic psychology student wanting to understand and to help people who were struggling. After four years, I left the university with a Bachelor's degree and some serious concerns about the legitimacy of current psychology. The political nature of who gets to decide what constitutes "normal" and "deviant" behavior, and the judgments of disorder that are based on these concepts, went almost entirely unacknowledged within the field. Although I had thought of psychology as fairly benign compared to psychiatry because of its focus on methods that do not involve drugs, I became disturbed by the undeniable connections between psychology, psychiatry, and psychotherapy—a constellation that has been broadly termed and critiqued as the psy-complex (Parker 2014). Although the fields constituting the psy complex differ from one another in philosophy and approach, they legitimize and propagate the same concepts, definitions, and "boss texts," thereby helping to strengthen one another despite their differences.

Toward the end of my schooling in psychology, I learned about the Cold War Era psychological experiments in Canada that have since been linked to the development of current Western military torture. I found this line of research, which highlights the connections between the field of psychology

E. Gold (✉)
Department of Leadership, Higher and Adult Education; OISE,
University of Toronto, Toronto, Ontario, Canada
e-mail: golde84@gmail.com

© The Editor(s) (if applicable) and The Author(s) 2016
B. Burstow (ed.), *Psychiatry Interrogated*,
DOI 10.1007/978-3-319-41174-3_11

and the development of torture, deeply troubling. Even though most of the critiques of the research on torture have focused on its military funding, these psychological experiments were funded as well by "mental health" organizations—thus my decision to investigate further and to write this chapter.

In this chapter, I explore the case study of Dr. John Zubek, a prominent psychologist at the University of Manitoba who was considered a leading world expert in the psychological development of torture techniques. A historical tracing of the organizations that funded Zubek's research as well as their funding mandates is followed by an institutional ethnography (IE) tracing of the role of ethical regulatory bodies in his research. A discussion of the implications of torture in military and psychiatric settings concludes the chapter.

Here traditional historical research (the majority of the chapter) is combined with IE. There are two IE components. One is the disjuncture—and to be clear, I am identifying the shock of what I was starting to uncover as a young psychology student as a disjuncture, in addition to what I am still uncovering. The other is precisely how the ethical regulating bodies worked so as to construct Zubek's research as ethical.

Background

In the early 1960s, a young undergraduate student at the University of Winnipeg's psychology department, Gordon Winocur, took a course taught by the department's head, Dr. John Zubek. Drawn to Zubek's dynamic lecturing style, Winocur soon became a research assistant in Zubek's prestigious lab. "We were encouraged to think this was groundbreaking research" (Rosner 2010, p. 33), Winocur recalls, and, in hopes of building a career under the prominent Chair of the psychology program, he volunteered to be one of the first participants to undergo a new experimental condition. Winocur entered a "coffin-like" box where his arms and legs were fastened with straps and his head was secured on three sides (Rosner 2010). Although the experiment was set to last 24 hours, Winocur lasted but 90 minutes in this condition, recalling: "It was horrible, really uncomfortable. If you have any latent claustrophobia, it's going to come out" (Rosner, p. 33).

After his participation, Winocur began to realize that Zubek's research agenda was something other than building theoretical understanding, stating, "[t]he major question was how well people reacted to this kind of treatment and what kinds of changes there were in perceptual and cognitive functions, things that might be useful in developing interrogation techniques" (p. 33). By "this kind of treatment," Winocur is referring to Zubek's 15 years of sensory deprivation and immobilization research, where more than 500 University of Manitoba students were subjected to experiments aimed at preventing them from having any sensory or perceptual input, as well as physical mobility. When Winocur declined Zubek's offer to do a graduate thesis under him, Zubek became infuriated, kicking Winocur out of his lab and threatening to kick him out of the entire psychology department (Rosner 2010).

Between the 1950s and 1970s, sensory deprivation research was a fascinating new area for psychologists and psychiatrists. This, the Cold War Era, was marked by anti-Communist paranoia and a push for "progress" in the West—whether scientific, military, or technological— and Western governments began funding research on an unprecedented scale (Noble 2011). It was during this era that interest grew in the newly termed idea of "brainwashing." In the early 1950s, psychologists began exploring how psychological methods could be used to modify and control behavior; an area of research that emerged as a significant military concern (Raz 2013).

In 1951, a secret meeting took place between several prominent scientists and members from the US Central Intelligence Agency (CIA) and the Canadian Defence Research Board (DRB). Dr. Donald Hebb, a psychologist at McGill University and a member of the DRB was present at this meeting and was the first to study sensory deprivation in the hopes of developing an understanding of brainwashing and of how ideas might be implanted into the "psyche" (Raz 2013).

Hebb experimented by placing McGill students into isolation chambers for several days at a time, where they wore translucent goggles, headphones that played constant white noise, cardboard or tubing over their arms, and gloves to prevent their sense of touch. What he found was that the students experienced vivid hallucinations and disorienting confusion. Hebb also began to loop repetitive audio tapes that suggested to the students that ghosts were real and science was not, with the purpose being to test whether ideas could be implanted into the students' "psyches."

Indeed, Hebb's results showed that in the weeks following their participation, the students became skeptical of science and developed interests in paranormal activity. They also remained extremely confused and intellectually stunted immediately following their period of isolation. In one document, Hebb noted that better results could be obtained if the students were kept in isolation for longer periods of 30–60 days; however, he could not justify keeping McGill students in a state of sensory deprivation for such long periods (Klein 2007; McCoy 2012). While Hebb hoped his subjects would remain in isolation longer, most of them dropped out of the study within the first few days and few made it a full week in isolation. Out of 22 subjects, four spontaneously informed Hebb that participating in his experiment was a form of torture (McCoy 2012).

Dr. Ewen Cameron, head of psychiatry at McGill, proceeded where Hebb felt he could not. Unlike his counterpart in the psychology department, Cameron saw no problem with keeping his un-consenting subjects in cruel and unusual states for months on end. Using psychiatric "patients" who did not know they were being experimented on (and therefore could not possibly give informed consent), Cameron sought to erase people's memories in the hopes of destroying their "problematic" personalities and rebuilding new ones upon what he expected to see as their blank slate of a brain. In this quest, Cameron repeatedly electroshocked his unfortunate "patients" at high doses, kept them in drugged stupors on massive amounts of psychiatric drugs, and much like Hebb, repeatedly played audio tapes for weeks and months at a time (Klein 2007; McCoy 2012). The McGill experiments provided the groundwork on which it was established that, at the very least, depriving people of their sense of space, time, and ability to think causes extreme confusion and disorientation and, at least temporarily, a lowering of one's intellectual, cognitive, and physical abilities.

Research on the history of sensory deprivation experiments has tended to focus on its military applications, particularly in the development of current Western torture techniques—a topic to which this chapter will return. However, at the time, psychologists took interest in what they believed would be the "therapeutic" applications of brainwashing. The theory, which speaks to psychological understanding at the time, was that "patients" who underwent sensory deprivation and brainwashing would be more susceptible to internalizing therapeutic messages and propaganda (Raz 2013). It was thought that brainwashing "patients" into a healthy "psyche" would help make psychotherapy a quicker and more efficient process (Raz 2013). Essentially, psychologists believed that successful therapy was contingent on the client internalizing the "therapeutic messages" they were receiving externally.

As a former psychology student, I found this line of reasoning disturbing; so I decided to check my first-year psychology textbook to identify some general goals of the field. In their introductory textbook, *Psychology*, Gleitman et al. (2004) state that psychology is "a field of inquiry that is sometimes defined as the science of the mind, sometimes as the science of behavior. It concerns itself with how and why organisms do what they do" (p. 3). A seemingly noble goal, to better understand the mind and behavior of animals including humans, the field of psychology has flourished with various theories to explain the mind and behavior, so-called deviance and psychopathology, and a variety of treatments and therapies to help people overcome their struggles (Gleitman et al. 2004). However, any field of study that concerns itself with understanding the "psyche" and behavior of humans is inherently vulnerable to straying from its stated goals. As can be seen by the interest of military intelligence in sensory deprivation research, the goal of understanding the mind and behavior of humans is susceptible to manipulation from special-interest groups with differing agendas.

The ties between psychology and the military have been documented by historian Ellen Herman, who argues that the Cold War "advanced psychological knowledge production on all the various fronts that constituted the psychological enterprise," which included the development of psychology, as cited in Kinsman and Gentile (2010), as an

> ...administrative discipline specializing in testing and classification; as a "helping profession" advancing psychotherapeutic techniques; and as a behavioral science devoted to investigating human motivation and action for the purposes of understanding, prediction, and control. (p. 173)

The field's claim of being able to predict personality and behavior was understood as increasingly important during the Cold War, particularly for dealing with *enemies* who were not always obvious (Kinsman and Gentile 2010). The threat of Communism infiltrating Western citizens frightened the governments of the West, a fear that was propagated to the general public; and the idea of enemies hiding in plain sight added to the paranoia of the era.

Dr. John Zubek, the prominent psychologist and world leader in sensory deprivation experiments, accepted a position as an assistant professor at McGill University in 1950—at first studying the behavior of rats under a variety of experimental conditions, but later moving on to human subjects and assisting Hebb in his sensory deprivation work. Although Zubek later denied being involved in Hebb's lab, documents and correspondences in his archives show otherwise (Rosner 2010; McCoy 2012). In 1953, Zubek accepted a position as the head of University of Manitoba's psychology department. In 1958, he was invited to join the Human Resources Research Committee of the DRB and the next year, Zubek started receiving DRB funding and began conducting his own sensory deprivation experiments on an unprecedented scale (Raz 2013).

Like Hebb, Zubek used university students, paying them for their participation. Where Hebb felt ethically limited to confine his subjects for periods no longer than several days, Zubek was on a mission to discover how long his subjects could last in varying states of suspended animation. So eager was Zubek to push the boundaries that he was the first to spend 10 full days immobilized in his sensory deprivation tank, experiencing hallucinations, a loss of motivation, and an inability to concentrate on anything intellectual (Rosner 2010). With financing from the University of Manitoba and the National Research Council of Canada (NRCC), Zubek set out to build the largest sensory deprivation lab in Canada—a goal he accomplished in 1968.

Between 1959 and 1974, more than 500 students underwent one of several of Zubek's agonizing experimental conditions for up to 14 straight days at a time, with a high percentage of them dropping out of the experiment within the first 12 hours. All of Zubek's experiments had a high dropout rate, generally ranging from one-third to three-quarters of participants leaving the experimental conditions early. Like Winocur, Zubek's subjects described their experience as grueling and uncomfortable, with many citing their participation as provoking intense anxiety, a loss of self, and, like Zubek, an inability to concentrate (JZ Collection, UMA, Box 6, Folder 12, Application for Mental Health Project 10/11/63). Even though Zubek theorized that the effects caused by his experiments were temporary, neither he nor Hebb reported any follow-up treatment and there is no way of knowing whether the trauma of participating in these experiments resulted in lasting damage (McCoy 2012).

For the first five years, Zubek's experiments resembled Hebb's, with students put into soundproofed sensory deprivation tanks and subjected to one of two main conditions. Some were placed in a sensory deprivation condition in a dark tank that prevented vision and had to wear noise-canceling headphones and special gloves to inhibit their ability to interact with their body and the environment (JZ Collection, UMA, Box 6, Folders 7–9). Here students stayed in complete silence, darkness, and isolation for up to two weeks. In the perceptual deprivation condition, subjects entered the tank with a fluorescent light shining through its contours, providing constant bright lighting but wore goggles preventing any patterned vision, and they were subjected to constant white noise through speakers placed by their heads, with their sense of touch blocked in the same manner as in the sensory deprivation condition (JZ Collection, UMA, Box 6, Folders 7–9).

The students who entered Zubek's sensory and perceptual deprivation lab had counted on filling their weeks of isolation by planning papers and presentations and thinking about their schoolwork. They found themselves, however, unable to concentrate on anything for the entire duration of their participation—an effect that added greatly to their experience of intense stress throughout the ordeal. They also described feeling cognitively and intellectually stunted as well as physically pained—findings that were validated through the battery of testing subjects were given before, during, and after the experiment. Trial after trial produced similar results, with high dropout rates, several hallucinations, and some students describing their experiences as highly stressful (JZ Collection, UMA, Box 6, Folders 7–9).

Over the years, Zubek began to suspect that maybe it was not the sensory and perceptual deprivation that was responsible for his dramatic findings; maybe it was being immobilized in a recumbent position for prolonged periods of time that was causing his subjects such intense discomfort. Throughout his research, Zubek noticed that the results from control subjects who merely stayed in the isolation tank without experiencing sensory or perceptual deprivation were largely similar (albeit less statistically significant) to the results with the experimental subjects. In 1964, Zubek introduced the particularly excruciating immobilization branch of his experiments. Subjects tested under this condition did not have constant bright lights and white noise in their environment, nor did they undergo the isolation of complete darkness and silence. For the most part, these subjects maintained their usual levels of sensory input (given that they were living in a laboratory). However, despite there being no interference with their ability to sense and perceive, only 8 out of 40 of the first exploratory subjects were able to tolerate this condition for a full 24 hours, with the majority dropping out, as Winocur did, in the first two hours (JZ Collection, UMA, Box 6, Folders 12–15).

In the immobilization condition, subjects entered a "coffin-like" box built especially for these experiments and had their legs strapped down and their arms tied to their sides, with their heads secured into position on three sides. The students stayed strapped in the coffin, without breaks, for as long as they could tolerate it—up to 24 hours. Considering that subjects reacted so strongly to this experimental condition, Zubek was surprised to find that no statistically significant intellectual impairments showed up in the testing of the eight subjects who lasted the full day. He theorized that the physical pain experienced by the students may have kept them more mentally alert and that "[p]ositive results might have occurred if a longer but less severe condition of immobilization had been employed" (JZ Collection, UMA, Box 6, Folder 12, Application for Mental Health Project 10/11/63, p. 5).

It seems, by this statement, that Zubek considered the presence of intellectual impairment a "positive" result. He also tried to identify physiological and cognitive differences between subjects who could tolerate the experimental conditions for the full duration and those that he termed "the quitters." Although he found no cognitive or intellectual differences between the groups, Zubek did find that those unable to tolerate the experimental conditions had lower baseline levels of noradrenalin (JZ Collection, UMA, Box 6, Folders 7–9).

On a quest for "positive results," Zubek adjusted the experimental condition, adding bathroom and meal breaks and unstrapping subjects for nine hours while they slept (although they were still unable to move) at the same time extending the length of the experiment to two weeks in order to test whether intellectual impairments would occur. Under the adjusted conditions, a higher percentage of subjects were able to live through the full two weeks of immobilization, and Zubek was able to achieve the "positive" results he was seeking—that is, he was able to produce *statistically significant intellectual impairments in his subjects* (JZ Collection, UMA, Box 6, Folders 12–15). These students described experiencing increasingly vivid and complex dreams, body-image distortions, a loss of contact with reality, distortions in time, intellectual inefficiencies, and bizarre thoughts along with a slew of physical discomforts that one might imagine to result from two weeks of ongoing physical immobilization. Hallucinations, while present, were rare.

The physical, cognitive, and intellectual impairments continued for weeks after the experiments ended, lessening over time (JZ Collection, UMA, Box 6, Folders 12–15). There is something deeply unsettling about experiments aimed at producing such dramatic impairments in subjects, which leaves one to wonder how such blatantly unethical research could openly take place in a respected university psychology department. The disjuncture of how students came to be tortured in the name of psychological progress is our entry point.

What Is Torture?

In 1984, the United Nations Convention Against Torture (CAT) introduced the following definition of torture:

[A]ny act by which severe pain or suffering, whether physical or mental, is intentionally inflicted on a person for such purposes as obtaining from him or a third person information or a confession, punishing him for an act he or a third person has committed or is suspected of having committed, or intimidating or coercing him or a third person, or for any reason based on discrimination of any kind, when such pain or suffering is inflicted by or at the instigation of or with the consent or acquiescence of a public official or other person acting in an official capacity. It does not include pain or suffering arising only from, inherent in or incidental to lawful sanctions. (Article 1; see http://www.un.org/documents/ga/res/39/a39r046.htm)

Instrumental to this definition is the intention to inflict pain or suffering for a purpose—whether that purpose is to gain information, to punish, or to intimidate. The other necessary condition to be met in this definition is that such pain and suffering must be inflicted by, at the instigation of, or with the consent of a public official.

The enhanced military interrogations that have been shown to arise out of sensory deprivation research have long been criticized as torture (Rosner 2010; McCoy 2012; Raz 2013). Indeed, when considering the preceding UN definition, the military use of sensory deprivation findings to intentionally inflict pain and suffering on prisoners of war for the purposes of gaining information, confessions, or even for the purposes of punishing seems to meet the criteria for CAT's definition of torture. These acts are sanctioned by the military, an influential branch of most governments. For an in-depth discussion of sensory deprivation research and its links to military torture, see Klein (2007) and McCoy (2012).

Even though it can be reasonably argued that the sensory deprivation research of the Cold War Era is military torture, does this, the original research itself, fit the criteria for torture? In Zubek's research, mental pain and suffering was intentionally inflicted on subjects, with the goal of the experiments being to obtain physical, cognitive, and intellectual impairment. Did Zubek know that he was helping to develop torture techniques and subjecting his participants to what would amount to torture? Unclear. Nevertheless, the point is, whether Zubek knew he was developing torture techniques, what he certainly knew were the effects he was producing in his subjects—vivid dreams and hallucinations, intense anxiety and claustrophobia, physical pain, and a complete inability to concentrate. Zubek also knew that these results were present in the tests he gave to his subjects.

With this knowledge, as well as knowledge of the McGill experiments that preceded him, Zubek continued this line of experimentation for 15 years. This fits the criteria of intent outlined in the CAT definition. Note, the purpose of subjecting participants to these experiments was to extract information; not specific information held only by the subjects, but rather information about how humans react to such conditions. That said, there is one important caveat to bear in mind when considering Zubek's experiments—unlike the victims of military and other types of torture, his participants were technically free to leave the experimental conditions at any time. Doing this, however, could conceivably be made more difficult in a state of disorienting confusion and complex dreaming as well as the fact that students by virtue of being students were in a one-down position. This raises the question of how experiments on torture, at least partially for the purposes of being applied as military torture, could come to take place posing as "neutral" scientific research. Where were the ethical regulatory bodies to enforce research standards?

How Do Ethics Apply?

In 1959, the Canadian Psychological Association (CPA) adopted the Code of Ethics used by the American Psychological Association (APA) for a three-year provisional period, during which time they would consider revisions. The APA ethics standards were released for the first time in 1953 and, although the guidelines were led by the ethical questions posed by psychologists, there was still a lot missing—including clearly articulated ethical research standards. Largely, the first edition of the APA Code of Ethics left ethical dilemmas to the discretion of psychologists (Conway 2012).

Nevertheless, even with the lack of explicit ethical research standards coming from the CPA, the Nuremberg Code (1947/1949) had outlined a set of 10 standards that physicians must conform to when conducting experiments using human subjects. The Nuremberg Code established a new set of ethical medical behavior in the post-WWII era and was created as a reaction to the shocking "medical research" that was conducted by the Nazis on Jews, "queers," and other marginalized persons. The Code stresses the importance of obtaining informed consent from subjects and of the experimenter's responsibility to avoid research that is unnecessary or that causes subjects pain and suffering. Standards 2, 4, and 6 of the Nuremberg Code are as follows:

> 2. The experiment should be such as to yield fruitful results for the good of society, unprocurable by other methods or means of study, and not random and unnecessary in nature.
> 4. The experiment should be so conducted as to avoid all unnecessary physical and mental suffering and injury.
> 6. The degree of risk to be taken should never exceed that determined by the humanitarian importance of the problem to be solved by the experiment. (1947/1949)

These three standards in themselves highlight just how questionable Zubek's research was. In these experiments, Zubek essentially manipulated uncomfortable conditions to see how his subjects would react, with the hopes of producing physical and mental impairment—a direct violation of the Nuremberg Code.

Although that Code leaves a grey area when it comes to producing suffering during human experimentation, it requires justification, either by yielding "fruitful results for the good of society" or by taking risks that do not "exceed that determined by the humanitarian importance of the problem to be solved by the experiment." Arguably, were Zubek's experiments held to the standards of the Nuremberg Code, they would have been deemed unethical. The development of torture techniques does not seem to warrant the suffering Zubek's subjects were put through. The necessity of such experiments cannot be justified as a response to any immediate threat, but rather, at best, as a form of preparation for future defense. Can the development of torture be deemed fruitful for the good of society? It is highly questionable, but this seems to be the only viable result produced from Zubek's work.

With research aimed at studying the "psyche" and behavior of humans and other animals, high ethical standards in psychology that protect research subjects are critical. "Psychologists take the issue of research ethics very seriously, and virtually every institution sponsoring research—every college and university, every funding agency—has special committees charged with the tasks of protecting human and animal participants" (Gleitman et al., p. 32). It is now known that *no such committee* was developed at the University of Manitoba to oversee Zubek's research until 1966, seven years into the experiments (JZ Collection, UMA, Box 6, Folders 12–15). In Canada, it is the CPA that is tasked with providing ethical guidelines for psychologists as well as enforcement of their standards; however, as we already know, the CPA Code of Ethics provided no research standards during this time period.

In 1950, the CPA created a Committee on Ethics whose primary activity was to develop a Code of Ethics. Early on, the Committee decided to adapt the APA's ethics code, and it appears as though they did not meet for years at a time following this decision. In 1959, the year that Zubek's experiments began, the Chair of the Committee on Research Financing wrote to the CPA, stating: "If it is decided to continue the existence of this Committee, the Chairman asks to be relieved of the responsibility of keeping it in a state of suspended animation" (Conway, p. 44). That was the year that the CPA provisionally adopted the APA's "Ethical Standards for Psychologists," after which the Committee remained relatively inactive for years, seeming to seek and receive little feedback from its members (Conway 2012).

It was not until 1976, two years after Zubek's research ended, that the CPA added a section on ethics in the conduct of research on human subjects to its Code of Ethics, well after the Nuremberg Code (1947/1949) and the Declaration of Helsinki (see World Medical Association 1964) had published widely adopted international ethical standards (Conway 2012). The Declaration of Helsinki, though not a legally binding document, is the set of ethical standards that the University of Manitoba's President, H. H. Saunderson, claimed the university was abiding by (JZ Collection, UMA, Box 6, Folders 12–15). The declaration was released by the World Medical Association and provides a set of ethical standards for medical research involving human subjects.

In its original basic principles, Sections 3–5 of the Declaration of Helsinki state:

> 3. Clinical research cannot legitimately be carried out unless the importance of the objective is in proportion to the inherent risk to the subject.
> 4. Every clinical research project should be preceded by careful assessment of inherent risks in comparison to foreseeable benefits to the subject or others.
> 5. Special caution should be exercised by the doctor in performing clinical research in which the personality of the subjects is liable to be altered by drugs or experimental procedure. (JZ Collection, UMA, Box 6, Folder 14)

Particularly in regards to these three standards, it is questionable that Zubek's research passed the scrutiny of the Declaration of Helsinki, as claimed by President Saunderson. Having known the results of Hebb and Cameron's research at McGill University, Zubek should have been well aware that he was embarking on research aimed at altering the personality of his subjects, even if he believed that these alterations would be temporary. Furthermore, similar to the debatable adherence of Zubek's work to the Nuremberg Code, it is seriously questionable whether the development of torture techniques is of such great importance as to warrant the torture inflicted on Zubek's subjects.

Even though the goal stated by Gleitman et al. (2004) of taking research ethics very seriously in psychology sounds necessary and responsible, there is nothing to suggest that such ethical standards existed other than a vague deference to international standards and through the existence of committees that never met or produced any documents or policies. In other words, despite the fact that there was supposed to be ethical scrutiny of psychological research and practice in Canada during the Cold War Era, in Zubek's case, there never actually was. Figure 11.1 shows the sequence of actions and inactions that institutionally enabled Zubek's research. Note, the inactions of ethical regulatory bodies were just as instrumental to the continuation of this unethical research as the actions of the direct funders.

For its part, the University of Manitoba seemed content with the funding and accolades that Zubek's work was attracting. President Saunderson was happy to meet with Zubek's funders when they visited the campus, helping to arrange their accommodations and joining them for campus tours and lunches (JZ Collection, UMA, Box 6, Folders 7–9). When a funder inquired about the ethicality and thoroughness of informed consent, which appeared to be questionable in Zubek's research, Saunderson signed off on a letter dismissing

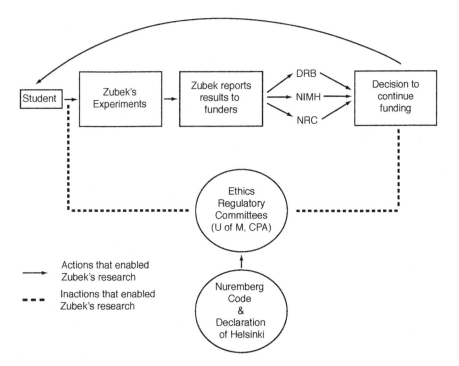

Figure 11.1 Cycle of actions and inactions that enabled Zubek's research.

concerns and questions and agreed to oversee the formation of a committee that would evaluate issues of ethicality and ensure the protection of subjects in Zubek's experiments. The minutes of the meeting show that it was decided that Saunderson should inform the funders that the university was abiding by the Declaration of Helsinki (JZ Collection, UMA, Box 6, Folder 14, Minutes of President's Committee 17/08/1967). Herein lies the beginning of an institutional fiction, which in essence constructs Zubek's work as ethical.

Although Gleitman et al. (2004) concede that in psychological research, "[d]ecisions about risk or deception are sometimes difficult, and the history of psychology includes many conflicts over the ethical acceptability of psychological studies," they assert that this only highlights the importance of a multidisciplinary supervisory committee tasked with protecting research subjects—a committee that in actuality seems to have done little if anything. The authors add:

> In addition, the protection of human and animal rights simply prohibits a number of studies no matter how much might be learned from them. We mentioned earlier that no experimenter would physically abuse research participants to study the effects of abuse. Likewise, no ethical investigator would expose participants to intense embarrassment or anxiety. (pp. 32–34)

In light of the conditions that were "ethically" experienced by Zubek's subjects, this statement reads as cynical at best. Essentially, a ghost committee was supposed to provide ethical guidelines as well as oversight and enforcement of those guidelines.

This committee, supposedly with the interests of Zubek's subjects at heart, was tasked with the responsibility of protecting the subjects from the agonizing experimental conditions as well as the cognitive, intellectual, physical, and physiological impairments they experienced as a result of participating in Zubek's studies. In reality, there is no indication that any of this happened. In IE terms, the ghost committees, much like Saunderson's letter, may be seen as an institutional fiction used to construct Zubek's work as ethical. This particular institutional fiction played a crucial role in creating the impression that Zubek's experiments had faced and passed ethical scrutiny and oversight when in reality, there is nothing to indicate this was the case.

In 1966, seven years after Zubek's research began and in response to ethical questions raised by the National Institute of Mental Health, the University of Manitoba, under the oversight of President Saunderson, set up its own ghost committee of Zubek's colleagues, selected by Zubek, who were tasked with evaluating the ethicality of his research and making recommendations where they saw fit. Much like the institutional fiction represented by the committees of the CPA, there is no reason to believe that this committee ever met, nor did any of its members express reservations or provide suggestions to Zubek at any point (JZ Collection, UMA, Box 6, Folders 12–15).

THE REALITY OF FUNDING

Materially, what enabled these experiments to actually happen and continue over the course of 15 years—besides the institutional pretence—was money. Without continuous funding, Zubek would have had no lab, no subjects, no assistants; nothing of what he needed to bring these experiments to life. Zubek's research was primarily funded through yearly grants from three organizations: the Defence Research Board, the National Research Council, and the US National Institute of Mental Health (NIMH). It is now known that during the Cold War, the CIA provided $25 million in funding for sensory deprivation experiments like Zubek's, which they funneled to the universities through the guise of other organizations. Whereas direct funding links have been made between the CIA and the Hebb and Cameron research at McGill University, such direct links have not been made in the case of Zubek (McCoy 2012; Rosner 2010). However, it is known that following the Permanent Joint Board on Defense (1940), military information was allowed to be freely exchanged between Canada and the USA (Stacey 1954). Canada likewise shared its military information with Britain and the DRB included members who were top US and British military personnel (Rosner 2010; McCoy 2012).

It was the National Defence Act (NDA 1950) that created and defined the Defence Research Board and its responsibilities. Section 53(1) of this Act defines the scope and functions of the DRB as follows:

> There shall be a Defence Research Board which shall carry out such duties in connection with research relating to the defence of Canada and development of or improvements in material as the Minister may assign to it, and shall advise the Minister on all matters relating to scientific, technical, and other research and development that in its opinion may affect national defence.

The Minister being referred to here is the Minister of Defence. The Act continues to define the makeup of the DRB and bestows on it the power and autonomy to create regulations and by-laws to govern its procedures and hire employees as they see necessary.

Sections 54 (c) and (d) of the Act state that the DRB may, with the approval of the Minister:

> (c) enter into contracts in the name of His Majesty for research and investigations with respect only to matters relating to defence; and
> (d) make grants in aid of research and investigations with respect only to matters relating to defence and establish scholarships for the education or training of persons to qualify them to engage in such research and investigations. (NDA 1950)

All of this would be paid for by Parliament as set out in Section 55 of the NDA. The Act does not elaborate on what constitutes research relating to matters of defense, but it does leave this decision at the discretion of the DRB. The Act also leaves the allocation of funds and the decision of how to disburse those funds among research projects up to the Board.

Of the three funding bodies, Zubek had the most intimate relationship with the DRB, which supported the sensory and perceptual deprivation branch of his experiments. At the time, the DRB was providing $30,000–50,000 in research funding per year, mostly to applied research outside of universities (Conway 2012). Of this, Zubek received $18,000–21,000 per year for the entire duration of the research, between 1959 and 1974, receiving a total of approximately $275,000 (JZ Collection, UMA, Box 6, Folders 7–9; McCoy 2011). Having spent two years on their Board and one as Chair for the DRB's Committee on Human Engineering, Zubek had developed a personal relationship with many of its members.

Zubek's membership in the DRB is an indication not only that the DRB was interested in his work but also that he probably had a type of insider's knowledge of what research initiatives the Board was likely interested. The DRB was immensely supportive of Zubek's work, even offering to provide him with military subjects for experimental conditions he felt too extreme for students; something Zubek occasionally did (JZ Collection, UMA, Box 6, Folders 7–9; Rosner 2010). Whether by conflict of interest or otherwise, as empowered by Sections 53–55 of the National Defence Act, the DRB came to fund Zubek's research for its entire 15 year duration.

The military relevance of these experiments seems to have been in testing how subjects would react to prolonged periods of isolation as well as sensory and perceptual deprivation and whether the intellectual, cognitive, physical, and physiological impairments that resulted from these conditions could be shown on a battery of tests. According to funding applications and progress reports, Zubek claimed the relevance to defense in these studies was counterintelligence against the Russian brainwashing of North American soldiers (the same justification as Hebb's). He also claimed his research would be relevant to the conditions faced by astronauts during space travel, a line of inquiry that largely falls outside of the mandate of the DRB (JZ Collection, UMA, Box 6, Folders 7–9).

Despite his collegial relationship with the DRB, the tides had started to shift for Zubek by the late 1960s. Although subjects were made to agree to keep their experiences in Zubek's lab confidential, word of former subjects' unusual and highly uncomfortable experiences in the lab got out and when a direct link was made between Zubek's research and new torture techniques being employed by the British military in Belfast, students at the University of Manitoba began protesting against Zubek's experiments (Rosner 2010; Raz 2013). At first, archival letters suggest, he believed that these protests would quietly disappear but, in reality, the students' grievances grew louder with time. For his part, Zubek defended his work, stating that "results can be used for wrong purposes and over this we as scientists have little to no control" (Rosner, p. 35). By relinquishing responsibility for the applications of his experiments, Zubek seems to be arguing that he was merely advancing the field of science in order to distance himself from the political interests intertwined within his experiments.

By 1971, Zubek had fallen out of favor not only with University of Manitoba students but also with his former ally, the DRB. After a review of his 12 years of sensory deprivation experiments, the Board recommended cutting or ending Zubek's funding, suggesting that his work was not making any notable advances in knowledge, was not leading to theoretical progress, and was of questionable quality. In a letter to Board member Dr. A. H. Smith defending himself against the review's findings, Zubek argued that the requirement of his research that subjects live in the laboratory added significantly to its defense applicability and that his development of measures that could predict which subjects would be unable to tolerate sensory deprivation had direct defense relevance (JZ Collection, UMA, Box 6, Folder 7, letter to A. H. Smith, 12/07/1971).

In the same letter, Zubek asked the DRB to continue his funding until 1974, the year that his grant from the NRCC would end, citing his 12-year record of "academic excellence," that he is a world leader in the sensory deprivation field, and the fact that his "productivity and its Defence relevance has never been an issue" (Letter to Smith, p. 4). Zubek concluded the letter by asking Smith to bring it to the attention of the highest levels of the DRB, as without their continued funding, he may be forced to close down his lab and continue his research "south of the border" (p. 6). According to archival documents, the DRB agreed to fund him until 1974, with Zubek's assurance that he would not reapply for DRB funding unless asked to do so (JZ Collection, UMA, Box 6, Folders 7–9).

The National Research Council of Canada was brought to life through the Research Council Act (1917) as a reaction to the shortcomings of Canada in advancing the fields of science and technology during WWI. After being created, it set up bursary and grant programs to assist with civilian science and technology research and also was responsible for advising the Canadian Cabinet on matters of science and industrial research. In 1924, a revision of the Research Council Act set up the NRCC as a corporation, giving it a full-time president and autonomy to control its expenditures and hire its own personnel. During WWII, the NRCC played an important role in Canada, essentially having a monopoly over knowledge in key sectors of science and technology (Smithsonian Institution, 2014). During this time, the NRCC also became heavily involved in military research, focusing much of its energy and resources on helping the war effort (Conway 2012). During the Cold War, the NRCC transitioned back to being responsible for civilian research, with military research falling under the jurisdiction of newly created organizations such as the DRB (Conway 2012). According to archival documents, the NRCC played a supporting role to the DRB, supplementing Zubek's budget with a six-year annual grant when he lost funding from the NIMH (JZ Collection, UMA, Box 6, Folders 3–5).

During the 1950s, the NRCC Committee on Applied Psychology was providing $15,000–25,000 per year in funding to psychology research; much like the DRB, mostly to research outside of universities (Conway 2012). In 1968, the NRCC provided Zubek with a one-time grant of $110,000 to build a new sensory deprivation lab at the University of Manitoba—the largest lab of its kind in Canada and one of the largest in the world. Their yearly contribution to Zubek's work was approximately $13,000 between 1968 and 1974—a large portion of their yearly budget but still the smallest contribution of the three main funders (JZ Collection, UMA, Box 6, Folders 3–5).

The NIMH is a US organization created by the National Mental Health Act (NMHA 1946). Section 2 of this Act explains that its purpose "is the improvement of the mental health of the people of the United States through the conducting of researches, investigations, experiments, and demonstrations relating to the cause, diagnosis, and treatment of psychiatric disorders." The Act goes on to define psychiatric disorders as including "diseases of the nervous system which affect mental health." This definition is problematic not only because of its vagueness but also because no physiological evidence of the existence of any psychiatric disorder has ever been shown (Burstow 2015).

Section 11 of the NMHA, the section that introduces the creation of the National Institute of Mental Health, sets aside $7.5 million for the erection and equipment of facilities, laboratories, and hospitals that would come to constitute the NIMH. Why I am introducing this Institute at this time, is that interestingly, NIMH funded Zubek's immobilization experiments—an experimental condition that was shown to be "more effective" than sensory deprivation seemingly because it was found intolerable by 80% of its initial participants (JZ Collection, UMA, Box 6, Folders 12–15).

In his initial funding application, Zubek cited the applicability of his research to understanding the effects of immobilization to patients in a "hospital setting;" to exploring the possible "retardation" that occurs to babies who are swaddled; and, interestingly, to "add to our basic store of knowledge concerning the role of kinesthetic-proprioceptive stimulation in the maintenance of *normal* behavior" (emphasis added; JZ Collection, UMA, Box 6, Folders 12, Application for Mental Health Project, 10/11/63, p. 5). The first two applications cited by Zubek seem largely irrelevant and outside the scope of the NIMH mandate which is "addressing diseases of the mind" (NMHA 1946). Regardless, the NIMH provided Zubek with approximately $30,000 per year in funding between 1964 and 1967, when the organization began to fund only US research (JZ Collection, UMA, Box 6, Folders 12–15). In total, Zubek received upwards of $90,000 from the NIMH (McCoy 2012). Although this is the only organization to fund Zubek's research with no overt military ties, the NIMH's support alerts us to the presence of another special-interest organization looking to build "relevant" knowledge on conditions experienced by subjects as intensely uncomfortable and anxiety invoking.

Although the DRB, NRCC, and NIMH were all brought into existence by law, they maintained the autonomy to make decisions about which research projects were relevant to their fields and to what extent each decidedly relevant project would receive funding. In other words, each organization allocated research funds as they saw fit and in the case of John Zubek, they all decided that this research was of relevance to their mandate. Figure 11.2 shows the organizations that monetarily supported Zubek's work over the years. Even though Zubek (at least publicly) relinquished responsibility over how his research was used by these special-interest organizations, their ongoing funding suggests that these bodies believed that Zubek's studies would help advance their respective causes. The presence of these organizations speaks to the different agendas behind Zubek's work.

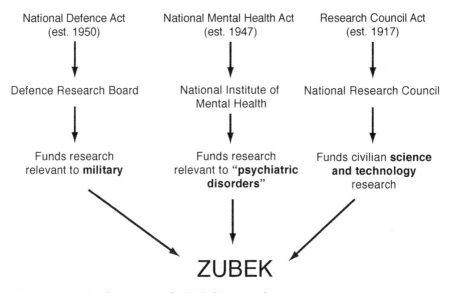

Figure 11.2 Funding sources for Zubek's research.

Discussion

It was argued earlier that Zubek's experiments meet the criteria of the definition of torture. Students were knowingly and purposefully placed into experimental conditions that caused them pain and suffering. These experiments were sanctioned by the University of Manitoba, and the ethical regulatory body for the field of psychology, the CPA, never stepped in, thus creating the illusion that Zubek's work met ethical standards. Zubek's research was directly linked to military torture through one nagging question that he could never escape—if not torture, what was the DRB's interest in funding this research? This telling link led to the demise of John Zubek who, shortly after losing all funding, was found floating in Winnipeg's Red River; a death that was ruled a suicide (McCoy 2012).

Nevertheless, little research has questioned the interests of Zubek's other major funder—the US National Institute of Mental Health. We now know that this research was linked to the development of current military torture techniques—methods that cause pain and suffering without inflicting direct physical violence on the victim. It seems worthwhile to ask here: What is the overlap between the development of military torture and the burgeoning field of mental health? If not torture, what was the NIMH's interest in funding this research?

Recalling the actual experiments, the National Institute of Mental Health primarily funded the immobilization branch—the most intolerable condition in Zubek's repertoire. Although most research has focused on the sensory deprivation aspect of the experiments, it was the immobilization that most subjects were simply unable to bear. This condition—having one's head and limbs strapped while in a recumbent position, even with normal levels of sensory input—was experienced as excruciating, with only one-fifth of the research subjects continuing their participation until the end. Not only was this condition intolerable to most participants, but it also produced intellectual stunting, a loss of contact with reality, and severe distortions in participants' perceptions (JZ Collection, UMA, Box 6, Folders 12–15). It is worth noting that Zubek's immobilization condition bears a striking and eerie resemblance to the common practice of physical restraint in mental health settings.

Until the late eighteenth century, those deemed "mentally ill" were chained in dungeons and cells. The use of physical restraint following this period was considered *humane* because the restraints used were now covered in cloth or leather; and the use and duration of restraints became contingent on the written order of the physician in charge (Meyer 1945). It is clear that the use of physical restraint in psychiatric contexts long predates Zubek's experiments, and whereas these two phenomena share many parallels, there is no historical link between them. However, it is interesting to note that actions that constituted psychiatric treatment, whether knowingly or not, were used to develop military torture techniques. Until relatively recently, physical restraints in psychiatric settings were viewed as a form of treatment with "patients" being kept immobilized, much like in Zubek's studies, for indefinite periods. Unlike Zubek's subjects, however, individuals who are being forcibly restrained in a psychiatric context do not enjoy the option of deciding whether they consent to being restrained and how long this period of restraint should last.

The use of physical or mechanical restraints in psychiatric institutions is largely unregulated and left at the discretion of doctors and hospital staff, with no requirements that restraints only be used when there is a serious threat of injury (Saks 1986). It appears as though, even now, a "patient" can remain physically restrained indefinitely; roughly comparable to Zubek's most intolerable condition, where only 8 of 40 subjects were able to last 24 hours. While the maximum period that people can be *legally* physically restrained for is generally 24 hours, doctors and hospital staff can get around this limitation by unstrapping a person for several minutes per day (Mion et al. 1996).

Although the Acts governing the use and duration of physical restraint vary among states and provinces, what becomes clear in comparing several of them is a general lack of guidance and oversight in cases where restraint is used. In Maryland, the state housing the National Institute of Mental Health, psychiatric "patients" can be restrained up to 24 hours, after which a face-to-face evaluation with a physician must be conducted to determine whether continuation of restraint is "appropriate." As stipulated by Section 10.21.12.09 D (2) of Maryland's Mental Hygiene Regulations (n.d.), restraint can only continue for periods longer than 48 hours "if the treating physician's documented clinical opinion is that the patient, if released from restraint, would continue to present a danger to self or others or would present a *serious disruption to the therapeutic environment*" (emphasis added). What constitutes a serious enough disruption to the therapeutic environment to subject a person to torture? Ultimately, that decision is left at the discretion of the physician; however, it is conceivable that "patients" who disagree with their "treatment" or ones who are disliked by staff may become unfairly targeted for restraint.

For comparison, the Commonwealth of Massachusetts has far more detailed regulations on the use of physical restraint in psychiatric institutions. According to the Massachusetts Mental Health Act (n.d.), orders of restraint can be given for a maximum of three hours, with the option of a three-hour continuation. After six hours, the use of restraint can be renewed by a physician who must document the reason restraint was used and the reason it "needs" to be continued. In Manitoba, the province where Zubek conducted his research, restraint is still considered a form of psychiatric treatment. The Manitoba Mental Health Act (2014) does not set time limits on the use of restraint, but simply states that "patients" may be restrained to prevent harm to themselves or others. The Ontario Mental Health Act (1990) is similar to that of Manitoba and both provinces require documentation, including a description of the means of restraint used, a statement of the duration or expected duration of restraint, and a description of the behavior that "required" restraint or continuation of restraint.

Essentially, regardless of jurisdiction, a person can be physically restrained for 23.9 hours out of every day (if not, in some places, continuously), through the written evaluation of a physician. It is also worth mentioning that people can be chemically restrained through the use of psychiatric drugs forever without any break; an important and related form of restraint deserving of intense ethical scrutiny.

In a report for the Joint Commission on Accreditation of Health Care Organizations, psychiatrist Peter Breggin (1999) defines "restraint" as:

> [T]he use of force or the threat of force for the purpose of controlling the actions of a person. Restraint includes a broad range of activities such as the use of "take downs," "therapeutic holding," and other bodily interventions; isolation rooms; strait jackets and four-point restraints; and neuroleptic drugs and other central nervous system depressants. The definition of restraint can also be broadened to include any restriction on the individual's freedom to reject a specific treatment or to leave the facility or setting. In this regard, involuntary treatment of any kind should be viewed as a form of restraint.

Despite centuries of practice in various forms, there remains no reason to believe that physical restraint is effective as a psychiatric treatment or as a method of subduing "patients" who are deemed unruly in this setting (Mion et al. 1996). Not only has the efficacy of physical restraint never been established, but its use has been directly linked to serious injuries and death. While physically restrained, people have died from strangulation and suffered limb injuries and skin trauma (Moss and La Puma 1991). Yet, learning and practicing methods of physical restraint are still among the first bit of training most new mental health workers receive, particularly in residential and hospital settings. By framing restraint as self-defense, or keeping the peace in the ward, or even helping to calm down a "patient" who is upset, workers routinely perpetrate this form of violence against those they are tasked with helping (Burstow 2015).

As noted by Moss and La Puma, in The Hastings Report, "the psychological consequences of humiliation and loss of dignity [suffered by individuals who are physically restrained] can lead to depression, a paradoxical increase in agitation, and behavioral problems similar to the constellation of symptoms seen in torture-related syndromes" (p. 23). In other words, individuals who are forcibly physically restrained can show similar symptoms to people who have lived through torture. In light of this, it is possible that Zubek's immobilization studies would help inform the known side effects of physically restraining people. Zubek did find that physical exercise helped to mitigate some of the cognitive, intellectual, and physiological impairments caused by immobilization (JZ Collection, UMA, Box 6, Folders 7–9, pp. 12–15)—a finding that does not seem to have been implemented in any procedural way across institutions that practice physical restraint. Despite the fact that at first Zubek's immobilization studies might seem like a bizarre line of experimentation, this opens the door to a far bigger disjuncture—how could immobilizing "patients," a condition shown by Zubek to cause impairments to subjects' well-being and experienced as unbearable by the majority, be considered a legitimate method of psychiatry?

In a UN Special Rapporteur on Torture and Other Cruel, Inhuman or Degrading Treatment or Punishment, Juan Méndez (2013) states:

> [T]here can be no therapeutic justification for the use of solitary confinement and prolonged restraint of persons with disabilities in psychiatric institutions; both prolonged seclusion and restraint constitute torture and ill-treatment. … [M]edical treatment of an intrusive and irreversible nature, when lacking a therapeutic purpose or when aimed at correcting or alleviating a disability, may constitute torture or ill-treatment when enforced or administered without the free and informed consent of the person concerned. … Furthermore, deprivation of liberty that is based on the grounds of a disability and that inflicts severe pain or suffering falls under the scope of the Convention against Torture. In making such an assessment, factors such as fear and anxiety produced by indefinite detention, the infliction of forced medication or electroshock, the use of restraints and seclusion, the segregation from family and community, should be taken into account. (p. 7, 14, 16)

Throughout the report, Méndez refers to individuals who are the recipients of forced psychiatry as having "mental disabilities." Interestingly, Méndez focuses on the lack of informed consent and the fear and anxiety caused by forced psychiatry as factors qualifying this as torture. Yet, despite this special report, military torture continues to be more high profile, with relatively little attention paid to the torture that is systematically taking place in so-called mental health settings.

Human rights lawyer and psychiatric survivor, Tina Minkowitz, has long argued that restraint in a mental health services context (along with many other acts involved in forced psychiatry) constitutes torture under the CAT definition. When individuals live through the torture of forced psychiatry, their trauma is typically unacknowledged and largely unseen by society. Minkowitz (2015) states:

> [M]y colleagues have documented the kinds of suffering and the scope of harmful consequences of forced psychiatry in a person's life. The severity of our subjective experiences of pain and suffering needs to be acknowledged … too often we are disbelieved and our suffering is made to seem insignificant.

For her detailed argument of forced psychiatry as torture, see Minkowitz 2015.

In *The Myth of Mental Illness*, Thomas Szasz (1974) argues that psychiatry is a pseudoscience—one concerned with symbols and representations rather than with objective illness or disease that can be detected by medicine. In comparing neurology with psychiatry, Szasz states:

> Neurology is concerned with certain parts of the human body and its functions *qua* objects in their own rights—not as signs of other objects. Psychiatry, as defined here, is expressly concerned with signs *qua* signs—not merely with signs as things pointing to objects more real and interesting than they themselves. (p. 47)

In other words, psychiatry attempts to embody "diseases of the mind" as though this were an objective, biological disease that could be detected as concretely as something like high blood pressure, for example. Szasz argues that "mental illness" should be understood as a metaphor, distinguishing it from actual illness, which can be detected in the body using various medical testing.

Elaborating on this concept in her book, *Psychiatry and the Business of Madness*, Burstow (2015) asserts:

> Of course, the brain is an organ of the body; brains do have illnesses; accordingly, for centuries now biological psychiatrists have argued that "mental illnesses" are brain diseases whose physical-chemical markers are simply yet to be discovered. … [A]fter over a century of looking, and indeed after dedicating vast sums of money to such research, moreover with bald-faced assertions ever circulating, including from official sources, that schizophrenia, for example, has been "discovered" to be a brain disease, there is no proof whatsoever that a brain disease or any other disease underlies any of the current "mental illnesses." The fact that this is an institution that operates on conjecture and declaration rather than on proof, an institution that not just occasionally but routinely calls things diseases in the absence of observable physical markers, I would add, raises the question whether we are truly dealing with medicine here, at least in the modern sense of the term. Indeed, it raises the question of whether we are dealing with science at all. (pp. 13–14)

If "mental illness," the concept on which psychiatry has been built, can be understood only as a metaphor as opposed to a legitimate observable science, this casts serious doubts on the psy-complex, including the institution of psychiatry, its legitimacy, and its powers to enforce. For an in-depth discussion of these topics, see Burstow (2015) and Szasz (1974). For the purposes of this chapter, it is important to note that psychiatry is the only institution in the Western world with the power to indefinitely imprison those who have committed no crime and to paternalistically "treat" individuals against their will; both violations of basic human rights.

In Zubek's experiments, subjects were purposefully placed in conditions known to produce pain and suffering and they were placed in those conditions for the purpose of studying the effects of how humans react to the various situations. Although it may have been difficult for many subjects to end their participation because of the effects of the experiments (i.e., disorientation and confusion), they were technically free to leave at any time. For those imprisoned in similar conditions under forced psychiatry, there is no escape.

Concluding Remarks

Decades after the end of Zubek's research, there seems to have been no other viable knowledge produced aside from the effects of various methods of torture on human subjects. Although some attention has been paid to the links between this research and the development of current Western military torture techniques, little has been noted about the use of these torture techniques in psychiatric and other so-called mental health settings. The everyday violations and abuses of human rights occurring under the guise of psychiatric treatment remain largely unquestioned despite the fact that psychiatry has evolved as a false science, making false claims about diseases of the mind that cannot be physically founded.

Was Zubek's intention in conducting his research to inform the development and known effects of torture in military and psychiatric settings? The answer to this remains unclear, but also quite irrelevant. In a 1963 book, *Eichmann in Jerusalem*, Hannah Arendt introduced the concept of "the banality of evil"—the idea being that those who commit the most unspeakable acts in human history are not particularly evil individuals, but ordinary citizens that subscribe to the doctrines of their society (Arendt 1963). In other words, the greatest atrocities get carried out by regular people going about their everyday lives in a given context. While Gordon Winocur's experience in Zubek's lab helped him realize that something was not quite right with the experiments, Zubek's work went largely unquestioned for more than a decade. During that time, Zubek enjoyed his acclamation, publishing his research often, speaking at conferences, and rising to the stature of a leading world expert in sensory deprivation.

To conclude, I would pose this question: Are we as a society going about our everyday lives while complicit in everyday atrocities disguised as "help"?

REFERENCES

Arendt, H. (1963). *Eichmann in Jerusalem: A report on the banality of evil.* New York: Viking Press.

Breggin, P. R. (1999). *Principles for the elimination of restraint.* ISCPP Report. Retrieved from http://breggin.com/index.php?option=com_content&task=view&id=96

Burstow, B. (2015). *Psychiatry and the business of madness: An ethical and epistemological accounting.* New York: Palgrave Macmillan.

Conway, J. (2012). *A chronicle of the work of the CPA: 1938–2010.* Ottawa: Canadian Psychological Association.

Gleitman, H., Fridlund, A. J., & Reisberg, D. (2004). *Psychology* (6th ed.). New York: W.W. Norton & Company.

Kinsman, G., & Gentile, P. (2010). *The Canadian war on queers: National security as sexual regulation.* Vancouver: UBC Press.

Klein, N. (2007). *The shock doctrine: The rise of disaster capitalism.* Toronto: Alfred A. Knopf.

Manitoba, the Mental Health Act. (2014). *Manitoba laws.* Retrieved from the Government of Manitoba website at: https://web2.gov.mb.ca/laws/statutes/ccsm/m110e.php

Maryland, Mental Hygiene Regulations. (n.d.). *Subtitle 21.* Retrieved from the Government of Maryland website at: http://www.dsd.state.md.us/comar/subtitle_chapters/10_Chapters.aspx#Subtitle21

Massachusetts Mental Health Act. (n.d.). *Chapter 23.* Retrieved from the Commonwealth of Massachusetts website at: https://malegislature.gov/Laws/GeneralLaws/PartI/TitleXVII/Chapter123/Section21

McCoy, A. W. (2012). *Torture and impunity: The U.S. doctrine of coercive interrogation.* Madison: University of Wisconsin Press.

Mendéz, J. (2013). *Report of the Special Rapporteur on torture and other cruel, inhuman or degrading treatment or punishment.* United Nations General Assembly. Retrieved from http://www.ohchr.org/Documents/HRBodies/HRCouncil/RegularSession/Session22/A.HRC.22.53_English.pdf

Meyer, L. A. (1945). Restraint in the care of psychiatric patients. *The American Journal of Nursing, 45*(6), 445–450 Retrieved from http://www.jstor.org/stable/3416909.

Minkowitz, T. (2015). *Forced psychiatry is torture* [Web log comment]. Retrieved from http://www.madinamerica.com/2015/04/forced-psychiatry-torture/

Mion, L. C., Minnick, A., Palmer, R., et al. (1996). Physical restraint use in the hospital setting: Unresolved issues and directions for research. *The Milbank Quarterly, 74,* 3, 411–433. Retrieved from http://www.jstor.org/stable/3350307

Moss, R. J., & La Puma, J. (1991). The ethics of mechanical restraints. *The Hastings Center Report, 21*(1), 22–25 Retrieved from http://www.jstor.org/stable/3563342.

National Defence Act. (1950). *Acts of the Parliament, Dominion of Canada, Chapter 43.* Retrieved from the Lareau Legal website at: http://www.lareau-legal.ca/NDA1950.pdf

National Mental Health Act, US. (1946). *79th Congress, Chapter 538.* Retrieved from the Legis Works website at: http://legisworks.org/congress/79/publaw-487.pdf

Noble, D. F. (2011). *Forces of production: A social history of industrial automation.* New Brunswick: Transaction Publishers.

Ontario, Mental Health Act. (1990). *RSO 1990, Chapter M.7.* Retrieved from the Government of Ontario website at: http://www.ontario.ca/laws/statute/90m07#BK3

Parker, I. (2014). Psychology politics resistance: Theoretical practice in Manchester. In B. Burstow, B. LeFrancois, & S. Diamond (Eds.), *Psychiatry disrupted: Theorizing resistance and crafting the (r)evolution* (pp. 52–64). Montreal/Kingston: McGill-Queen's University Press.

Raz, M. (2013). Alone again: John Zubek and the troubled history of sensory deprivation research [Electronic Version]. *Journal of the History of Behavioral Sciences, 49*(4), 379–395.

Rosner, C. (2010). Isolation: A Canadian professor's research into sensory deprivation and its connection to disturbing new methods of interrogation [Electronic Version]. *Canada's History, August, 1,* 28–37.

Saks, E. R. (1986). The use of mechanical restraints in psychiatric hospitals. *The Yale Law Journal, 95*(8), 1836–1856 Retrieved from http://www.jstor.org/stable/796478.

Smithsonian Institution, Lemelson Center. (2014, July 23). *National Research Council of Canada fonds, 1916-1989.* Retrieved from http://invention.si.edu/national-research-council-canada-fonds-1916-1989

Stacey, C. P. (1954). The Canadian-American joint board on defence, 1940-1945. *International Journal, 9*(2), 107–124 Retrieved from http://www.jstor.org/stable/40197990.

Szasz, T. S. (1974). *The myth of mental illness: Foundations of a theory of personal conduct* (Rev. ed.). New York: HarperCollins Publishers Inc..

The Nuremberg Code. (1947/1949). In A. Mitscherlich & F. Mielke (Eds), *Doctors of infamy: The story of the Nazi medical crimes* (pp. xxiii–xxv). New York: Schuma.

World Medical Association. (1964). *WMA Declaration of Helsinki – Ethical principles for medical research involving human subjects.* Finland: Helsinki.

Zubek, J. Collection. (n.d.). *University of Manitoba Archives and Special Collections,* Elizabeth Dafoe Library, Winnipeg, Manitoba [cited as JZ Collection, UMA].

THE AFTERWORD

Where Have We Been?; What Have We Found Out?; Where Do We Go from Here?

Bonnie Burstow

We are fast approaching the end of a long and fascinating journey—one characterized by forays into several heretofore relatively unexplored nooks and crannies of the "mental health" system—the legal coordination of involuntary admission in Poland, for instance (Chapter 10), the little known but historically significant immobilization experiments which were tucked away at a western Canadian university (Chapter 11), and the everyday and strangely sanitized psychiatric stranglehold exercised over workers in the helping professions in the UK, Canada, and the US (Chapters 3 and 8). In the process, we have learned much about psychiatry and about the various realms over which it rules—directly or indirectly. And we have seen up-close critical details on how such ruling happens. Correspondingly, important discoveries have been made, important realities brought to light.

Examples are: In Canada minimally, ethical review processes are of little help in reining in even obviously problematic research, psychiatric or otherwise, for the monitoring body wields almost no power (Chapter 2). The coordination of lawyering in Poland relegates "mad lawyering" to the margins of legal work, thereby seriously jeopardizing the quality of representation (Chapter 10). International organizations that start off comparatively open slowly but surely become dominated by psychiatric constructs (Chapter 6). Correspondingly, psychiatric rule works in such a way that what might be construed as the "victims" of psychiatry in essence are forced into doing psychiatry's work for it (e.g., Chapter 5).

In this last regard, in one area after another, we have seen how texts and their activation come together with financialization, with media "hype," with the urgency of people's need for assistance, and with the restriction of resources to ones psychiatrically framed and controlled to create a veritable psychiatric stranglehold which willy-nilly leaves vulnerable individuals and their families, no matter how diligent or caring, succumbing to institutional capture. In essence, we have seen how folks are both seduced into and forced to actively embrace psychiatry. Witness, for example, the plight of the mother Sofia, as depicted in Chapter 5.

That said, it is beyond the scope of this book to articulate in any detail where solutions lie. To state the obvious, however, it is clear that psychiatry is integral to disjuncture after disjuncture, and as such, were the argument bolstered by solid medical evidence, a case could be made for dismantling the institution entirely (for a book which provides just such evidence and advances such a case, see Burstow 2015). Minimally, for those who do not go this far (and indeed, several of the contributors to this anthology do not), this much is obvious: Psychiatric tentacles are everywhere, with ever new tentacles constantly emerging. And so attacking the problem piecemeal is to a degree counterproductive. It would be a bit like lopping off one of the heads of the mythical Hydra, only to witness three more heads sprout up in its place. A signal once again pointing to the significance of abolition. At the same time it is clear that the stringent reining in of psychiatry in each of the areas explored is critical to attending to the problems which have surfaced—ergo, my commenting on them now.

To touch on a few of the areas and eke out the beginnings of directions, what if we reconfigured labor and government to accommodate support being given to workers without "input" from psychiatry and which was free of bureaucratic entanglements? A viable direction might include: Workers, in consort with management, figuring out problems and accommodations together; not obscuring but making visible problematic labor practices; the establishment of safe processes whereby workers could lodge complaints; and finally, to the extent possible, the introduction of worker self-rule, or, at the bare minimum, the flattening of hierarchical arrangements.

By the same token, what if instead of serving as entry points into "the mental health system," our schools were actively protected from psychiatric interference? Correspondingly, a plethora of nonmedical services, replete with choices, could be made available to the families of children in need of extra help—services, moreover, for which the receiving of a diagnosis is irrelevant. More fundamentally still, instead of being prisons where children are kept under control and constructed as a problem when they differ from a norm or cannot "keep up," what if our schools were turned into oases where kids are appreciated and nurtured in all their difference? Examples of concrete measures that might be taken are: minimizing the use of classrooms as a setting; the acceptance and even welcoming of rambunctiousness as a natural part of childhood; and making a critical part of the school curriculum an active valuing of the differences currently pathologized (for ideas on what this might look like, see Burstow 2015, Chapter 9).

More detailed avenues of redress for some of the problems uncovered to date include:

- With the reservations expressed at the end of Chapter 2 "a given," Canada's ethical review system as currently constituted should be changed so that the Secretariat can intervene in situations of extreme harm.
- Contrary to the highly problematic trend toward regulation, the helping professions, including those currently constructed as "regulated professions," should not so much be "regulating" their members as helping them do their work, providing support as needed. Nor should any organization have the right to compel a member to see a psychiatrist. Which is not to say that professions should not have standards. However, in instances of conflict, the possibility of unfairness and indeed oppression (e.g., racism, sexism, transphobia) could automatically be considered. Assistance—not control—and attention to local needs—not rule via extra-local texts—could be prioritized. Correspondingly, when difficulties arise, everyone could be involved in figuring out what happened and how it might be dealt with—with checks made for possible scapegoating, with the welfare of everyone considered, with everyone accepted as an expert on their own needs, and with no one's voice invalidated (consider in this regard how very differently Ikma's and Janet's lives might have played out—see Chapter 3—had they *actually been listened to*.
- Instead of diagnosing military personal with "PTSD" and subjecting them to brain-damaging drugs, we as a community could own our causal role in veterans' distress, pull back from armed conflict, and make a plethora of non-medical and empowering services and choices readily available to veterans (see Chapter 7).
- Rampant promotion/self-promotion by psychiatry and the multinational pharmaceutics could be actively discouraged, and misinformation and conflicts of interest rigorously constrained (see, for example, Chapter 5).

Of course, while progress and inroads can always be made, taking such measures in any major way would be contingent on a more general societal transformation, and, in effect, a new social contract (for one view of how society might be reconstituted, see Burstow 2015, Chapter 9). In short, another implication of this book.

A far more limited but nonetheless valuable contribution of this anthology is its multiple and tangible demonstrations of how useful IE is in making visible the link between everyday psychiatric operations and the concrete disjunctures that people face. In this regard, I stated in Chapter 1:

> The suitability of IE as an approach for interrogating psychiatry is demonstrable for psychiatry routinely causes disjunctures—indeed, horrendous disjunctures in people's everyday lives; it has both hegemonic and direct dictatorial power; and behind what we might initially see—a doctor or a nurse—lies a vast army of functionaries, all of them activating texts which originate extra-locally.

And indeed, so this anthology has demonstrated, whether the functionaries be members of military (Chapter 7) or everyday office managers (Chapter 9).

And this being the case, at this juncture I renew the invitation extended at the outset of our journey: Namely, as applicable, I invite those committed to psychiatric critique to add IE to their investigatory repertoire, likewise to conduct IE inquiries into psychiatry, whether it be delving further into areas touched on in this anthology or tackling ones largely or entirely absent from it—(e.g., specific disjunctures in specific Asian and African locales, the psychiatric colonization of Aboriginal communities, the progressive psychiatric colonization of the global south by the global north). By the same token, I renew my invitation to the IE community as a whole to once again place the mapping of psychiatric rule squarely on the IE agenda.

To leave the question of psychiatry for a moment, a more circumscribed relevance that this anthology holds is precisely for institutional ethnography work as a whole *irrespective of the type of disjuncture or ruling regime involved*. In this regard, it models a more open approach to IE—one that I hope will get taken up broadly. To be clear, while IE researchers certainly differ, there is a tendency in IE circles toward a type of rigidity or purism—not an uncommon development with modes of inquiry that have acquired a loyal following. Nowhere is this more clearly epitomized than in the response of one reader of this manuscript (anonymous) who stated unequivocally that in no way is this book's claim to be doing institutional ethnography supportable, that not a single chapter actually employs institutional ethnography, adding that besides that investigations into how the mental health regime is put together are sadly missing, the book actually precludes such an investigation.

Now this pronouncement notwithstanding, clearly the various contributors to this anthology *did* investigate how specific parts of the regime are put together, in the process mapping the everyday activation of texts. And as such, the critique will not hold. At the same time, unquestionably, we did depart from "purist IE" in a number of ways. While such a shift blatantly posed a problem for this particular scholar and doubtless will for certain others, in this very departure, I would suggest, lies a promising direction for IE.

To spell this out: For one, throughout, as investigators, we were clear about our respective positions. This stands in stark contrast with writing in quasi-neutral ways—something which, I would suggest, is problematic even epistemologically, for it is predicated on an epistemology of neutrality and what Harding (1991 and 2004) calls "weak objectivity," and as such, it inherently conflicts with standpoint theory. For another, instead of distinguishing sharply between IE and other methodologies, the contributors freely combine IE with other methodologies as helpful. Note in this regard the liberal use of critical discourse analyses in several of the pieces (e.g., Chapters 2 and 7) and of narrative analysis in others (e.g., Chapter 8). It has been suggested that institutional ethnography is in danger of becoming a regime of ruling in its own right (see, for example, Walby 2007). The more open approach to institutional ethnography herein epitomized could be one corrective.

That noted, admittedly, IE has often been combined with other approaches before—participatory research in particular (e.g., Smith and Turner 2014).

What is new here is the extent of it, the greater openness, the flexibility, which itself opens up fresh possibilities for inquiry. Approaches that combine particularly well with institutional ethnography and that I would especially encourage are critical discourse analysis on one hand and participatory research on the other, followed by dialectical materialism, narrative analysis, and grounded theory. No doubt there are researchers who would identify other combinations, and as long as they are backed by solid rationales and aid analysis, such innovations should be celebrated—not discouraged. Moreover, given that, as the savvy authors of Chapter 3 (A Kind of Collective Freezing-Out) so astutely point out, there are oppressions and ways of being oppressed that institutional ethnography per se does not pick up on well—everyday racism and sexism, for example—with some inquiries, I would add, it is critically important that other approaches, including ones not obvious, be folded in so that a fuller and more nuanced analysis emerges. Hence the potential value of such seemingly unlikely combinations as IE and heuristic research, not to mention phenomenology, with which, after all, IE inquiries inherently commence.

Now to date there has been an abundance of fusions of IE and participatory research and herein I find special promise. What is exciting about this combination is it further politicizes institutional ethnography, drawing on many of the strengths which initially surfaced with George Smith (1990). George Smith-style IE itself is intrinsically activist—hence the significance of Chapter 2 (the Burstow and Adam chapter). Even when not of an activist bent, however, that is, even when confrontation is minimal, the combination of IE with participatory research lifts IE out of the paradigm of the lone researcher positioned as *individually* able to achieve a viable standpoint—and it effectively reconfigures standpoint as a collective accomplishment. Hopefully, this anthology can help contribute to that participatory direction. Which brings me back to the narrower question of participatory research per se.

Participatory research with highly marginalized populations has become increasingly common over the decades, and generally when a project of this ilk is happening, something intrinsically worthwhile is transpiring. This notwithstanding, such projects commonly fall short of being emancipatory. What I find particularly promising about the Spirituality Psychiatrized project (Chapter 4) is that while involving a highly marginalized population, largely avoided is the comparatively top-down version of participatory research so often found in work with disenfranchised communities (for an example of what I am critiquing, see Yeitch's 1996 research). Note, every single member of the Spirituality Psychiatrized team, including Tenney, who serves as animator, hails from the marginalized population in question. And in no way does the participatory research operate as a for-profit business—a worrisome tendency that I will not be referencing but which I see emerging of late in the IE world.

Which brings me to one final point, one final contribution, one final invitation. I would remind readers that from the start of this project, one of its central purposes has been to help make IE skills available to the psychiatric survivor community. As such, it has in part been an exercise in capacity building. That work has clearly begun. In this regard, a large percentage of those who attended the IE workshops in the summer of 2014 were psychiatric survivors, gathering skills, adding to their repertoire. Additionally, the vast majority of the scholars who joined the workgroups in progress were survivors. Correspondingly, a third of the authors of this anthology are survivors. Moreover, as already noted, what is by far the largest team formed is comprised exclusively of survivors. So is one other. What adds to what is happening here is that after the completion of this manuscript Dorothy Smith held one of her legendary institutional ethnography workshops—and several survivors proceeded to take it.

The long-term relevance and viability of such a direction is, of course, for survivors themselves to determine. My hope, nonetheless, is that the spread of IE skills through this community continues. While the reining in of psychiatry is *all of our responsibility*, note, besides that IE can be an enormously useful tool, it is precisely with survivors and their work that much of the promise of overcoming psychiatry rule lies. My point here is that besides the fact that emancipation in the deepest sense occurs when people grapple with their own oppression, there is a special knowledge that survivors bring. Not that *all survivors have* or *any automatically have* what Hartsock (2004) calls an "achieved" standpoint, to be clear, but herein lies a community which for obvious reasons has privileged access to such a survivor standpoint.

Which brings us to a critical question—one stemming precisely from the "survivor-centric" nature of this project: Unquestionably, one of the great strengths of IE is the emphasis traditionally placed on the standpoint of the "hands-on" institutional worker. Critical though this dimension be, and indeed *pivotal* as front line workers' knowledge of institutional text-act sequences inevitably is, the question nonetheless arises: Why do IE researchers prioritize the location of and research done by institutional workers to *the extent* that we do? If the standpoint of the oppressed is less "partial" and less "perverse" (Hartsock 2004), what implication does this hold for those most oppressed by the system? To put this another way, insofar as we have a choice, why not give greater priority to the person or people experiencing the most horrific of the disjunctures, irrespective of whether or not they formally work for the organization, helping *them* become researchers, and in the process, achieving their "own" standpoint? Correspondingly, where the institution is medical (or pseudo-medical), why is the disjuncture picked so often that of the nurse? While certainly IE research arising from the standpoint of the front line institutional worker can produce stunning results (e.g., Diamond 2009)—and predictably, will continue to—should we not be trying to move at least somewhat more in the direction of the standpoint of the "patient"? Finally—and what might be called the "killer question" (and we surely need questions like this to be pondered by institutional ethnographers): What is lost, what sacrificed, when we assume that the standpoint of this front line worker, however beleaguered, however astute, and/or however caring, somehow "covers"—or adequately incorporates—the standpoint *or* the conundrum of the "patient"?

In ending, I would like to express my gratitude to all researchers who were part of this remarkable anthology project—whether you proceeded all the way to the submission stage or you walked with us but a short while. This is the kind of endeavor wherein everyone's involvement "mattered" and, indeed, continues to matter, irrespective of time spent. A special thanks additionally to those who sweated over revision after revision, not satisfied until the final "i" was dotted.

I would also like to express my gratitude to everyone who is in any way involved in the larger emancipatory anti/critical psychiatry project of which this anthology is a part—from activists demonstrating on the street; to inmates challenging their status of "incapable;" to parents who refuse to let their child be "assessed;" to nurses and other workers who vociferously object to their agency's slide toward greater and greater use of "diagnoses;" to authors who dare to write "subversively." Whatever the nature or the extent of your involvement and whatever your reason for it, you are part of one of the most important battles of the current era—a battle, indeed, which "defines" the current era. And you are liberation warriors—one and all.

Thank you and mazel tov, each and every one of you.

REFERENCES

Burstow, B. (2015). *Psychiatry and the business of madness: An ethical an epistemological accounting.* New York: Palgrave.

Diamond, T. (2009). *Making gray gold: Narratives of nursing home care.* Chicago: University of Chicago Press.

Harding, S. (1991). *Whose science? Whose knowledge: Thinking from women's lives.* New York: Cornell University Press.

Harding, S. (2004). Rethinking standing epistemology: What is "strong objectivity"? In S. Harding (Ed.), *The feminist standpoint theory reader* (pp. 127–140). New York: Routledge.

Hartsock, N. (2004). The feminist standpoint: Developing the grounds for a specifically feminist historical materialism. In S. Harding (Ed.), *The feminist standpoint theory reader* (pp. 35–53). New York: Routledge.

Smith, D. E., & Turner, S. M. (Eds.). (2014). *Incorporating texts into institutional ethnographies.* Toronto: University of Toronto Press.

Smith, G. (1990). Political activist as ethnographer. *Social Problems, 37*(4), 629–648.

Walby, K. (2007). On the social relations of research: A critical assessment of institutional ethnography. *Qualitative Inquiry, 11*(7), 108–130.

Yeitch, S. (1996). Grassroots organizing with homeless people: A participatory research approach. *Journal of Social Issues, 52,* 111–121.

Index[1]

[1] Note: Page numbers followed by 'n' denote notes.

© The Editor(s) (if applicable) and The Author(s) 2016
B. Burstow (ed.), *Psychiatry Interrogated*,
DOI 10.1007/978-3-319-41174-3